"In this inspiring book, Mark M. Smith blows the dust off the documents and monuments historians normally concentrate on in their efforts to reconstruct the past, and breathes new life into the sounds and textures, scents and sights that have shaped the consciousness of historical actors from antiquity to the present. *Sensory History* thus makes for sensational reading, and at the same time offers a critical take on the burgeoning literature in this dynamic new field of inquiry. Smith's history of the sensate is destined to precipitate a revolution in our understanding of the sensibilities that underpinned the mentalities of past epochs."
David Howes, *Concordia University*

"Who would ever have guessed that a book on the history of the senses – seeing, hearing, touching, tasting, and smelling – could be informative, thought-provoking, and, at the same time, most entertaining? Ranging in both time and locale, Mark Smith's *Sensory History* makes even the philosophy about the senses from ancient times to now both learned and exciting. This work will draw scholars into under-recognized subjects and lay readers into a world we simply but unwisely take for granted."
Bertram Wyatt-Brown, *University of Florida*

"A far-ranging essay on the history of the senses that serves simultaneously as a good introduction to the historiography. If one feels in danger of sensory overload from this growing body of scholarship, Smith's piece is a useful preventive."
Leigh E. Schmidt, *Princeton University*

"This is a masterful overview. The history of the senses has been a frontier field for a while now. Mark Smith draws together what we know, with an impressive sensory range, and encourages further work. A really exciting survey for established practitioners and ambitious students alike."
Peter N. Stearns, *George Mason University*

Sensory History

MARK M. SMITH

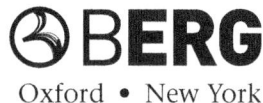
Oxford • New York

English edition
First published in 2007 by
Berg
Editorial offices:
First Floor, Angel Court, 81 St Clements Street, Oxford OX4 1AW, UK
175 Fifth Avenue, New York, NY 10010, USA

© Mark M. Smith 2007

All rights reserved.
No part of this publication may be reproduced in any form
or by any means without the written permission of
Berg.

Berg is the imprint of Oxford International Publishers Ltd.

Library of Congress Cataloging-in-Publication Data

Smith, Mark M. (Mark Michael), 1968-
   Sensory history / Mark M. Smith. — English ed.
       p. cm.
   Includes bibliographical references and index.
   ISBN-13: 978-1-84520-414-3 (cloth)
   ISBN-10: 1-84520-414-X (cloth)
   ISBN-13: 978-1-84520-415-0 (pbk.)
   ISBN-10: 1-84520-415-8 (pbk.)
  1. Senses and sensation—History. I. Title.
   BF233.S65 2007
   152.109—dc22

                                                                        2007035200

British Library Cataloguing-in-Publication Data

A catalogue record for this book is available from the British Library.

ISBN 978 1 84520 414 3 (Cloth)
      978 1 84520 415 0 (Paper)

Typeset by JS Typesetting Ltd, Porthcawl, Mid Glamorgan
Printed in the United Kingdom by Biddles Ltd, King's Lynn

www.bergpublishers.com

For Sophie and Bennett

Contents

Acknowledgements ix

Introduction: Of Sense and Non-Sense 1

1 Seeing 19

2 Hearing 41

3 Smelling 59

4 Tasting 75

5 Touching 93

Conclusion: Futures of Senses Past 117

Notes 133

Bibliography 157

Index 173

Acknowledgments

Careful eyes read parts or all of this book and discriminating ears listened to snippets of it in lecture form. A special thanks to Professor David Howes of Concordia University who read the manuscript and offered invaluable suggestions. David has been thinking carefully and creatively about the senses for a long time and I have benefited enormously from his pioneering work. He has my sincere thanks. My colleague, Professor Robert Herzstein, also offered encouraging remarks and judicious counsel and I thank him for his timely and thoughtful reading of the manuscript. An early version of the Conclusion was read by Professor Peggy Hargis of Georgia Southern University and by Professor Michael Grossberg of Indiana University, both of whom, from their quite different perspectives, offered very helpful criticism. I also asked Tara Crowe, my former student and now Exhibitions Administrator (Interpretation and Design) at London's Natural History Museum, to comment on parts of the book. Tara pressed me on issues relating to my critique of the use of sensory design in museums and I learned from her counsel.

At the University of South Carolina, Professor Tom Lekan, Professor Patrick Scott and, especially, my former colleague, Professor Karl Gerth, were kind enough to alert me to sources in their respective fields that I would have likely missed. Professor Richard Bauman of Indiana University, Professor Andrew J. Rotter of Colgate University, Professor Kathleen Hilliard of the University of Idaho, and Dr. Aaron Marrs of the Office of the Historian in Washington, D.C. did likewise and I remain in their debt.

I'm grateful to my graduate students – most notably David Prior and Mike Reynolds – who passed along sometimes priceless references. Particular thanks go to Jay Richardson and Rebecca Shrum for not only sharing information but for helping me think more carefully about the history of sight and vision. Jay's dissertation on the history of gaslight in the antebellum American South and Rebecca's on the history of mirrors in the United States promise to be important contributions to the literature.

Some of this book's arguments were delivered in lecture form as the Second Annual James Baird Lecture in the Department of History at the University of Southern Mississippi in 2006, as the keynote address of the Annual Meeting of the St. George Tucker Society in 2005, and as talks hosted by Rice University in Houston, the University of Illinois at Urbana-Champaign, the University of North Carolina, Chapel Hill, and at the Newberry Library in Chicago. I learned from the questions posed on each occasion.

Errors of commission and omission are, of course, mine alone.

Introduction
Making Sense of History

What Was, Is, and Is Not

This book tries to make sense of, well, the senses. It is a relatively short study of a very large topic. It traces the history of the senses from antiquity to the twentieth-first century, roams over dozens of countries and societies, takes seriously the history of seeing, hearing, smelling, tasting, and touching, and also considers how they operated in concert. It examines the importance of the senses to the principle developments of antiquity and the pre-Enlightenment era generally and it especially tries to understand their relevance to "modernity" – how, beginning in the West, principally in the seventeenth and eighteenth centuries, the senses informed the emergence of social classes, race and gender conventions, industrialization, urbanization, colonialism, imperialism, nationalism, ideas concerning selfhood and "other," to list the most obvious developments typically associated with the "modern" era.

I've aimed to be responsibly thorough but not catholic. It is not encyclopedic but, rather, something of an extended essay. It relies on my reading of a number of recent studies dedicated to sensory history and also on general treatments of any number of topics that I mined for nuggets of historical information about a particular sense. The past thirty years have witnessed an outpouring of historical work on the senses and this book canvasses a lot of it. The available work is uneven, however: there is less work on the importance of the senses in the pre-Enlightenment West than for the modern period and much more for the West – especially Europe and North America – than for the non-West. That unevenness is inevitably reflected in this book and it is likely that some of my conclusions will be revised as more work is done on these neglected areas. This is all to the good. I do not pretend to be exhaustive. I've missed some books, I'm sure, and decided against including other work. Rather, I've aimed to set the works I've chosen in dialogue, mainly in an effort to reframe an emerging historical conversation, especially among scholars who sometimes seem unaware that their colleagues in other fields and area specializations are working on similar problems.

In the course of the book, I introduce readers to the main works in a burgeoning area of scholarly inquiry and, in the process, argue a case. Its principal audience is the interested lay reader, especially students, but also scholars from any number of disciplines who would like to know something about the nature and content of historical work on the senses, a little about the historiography of sensory history (such as it is at the moment), and who also want examples of how the senses functioned and what they meant to various constituencies over a broad span of time and space. For those readers already familiar with histories of the senses, this book also offers an argument that, I hope, helps refine current frameworks for understanding the history of the senses. It argues that a prevailing association characterizing the so-called proximate senses of smell, taste, and touch as "premodern" is misleading and masks the ways in which non-visual senses proved central to the elaboration of modernity in a number of societies, especially in the West and North America but also in areas of Africa, South America, Australia, and China, too. Conversely, I also suggest that sight, while plainly important to the emergence of modernity, also functioned to iterate key aspects of pre-Enlightenment societies. Moreover, I claim that sight was not always the stable, rational sense either during or long after the invention and dissemination of print, the conventional historical pivot used by some observers – and accepted only in part in this book – to demarcate the supposed "great divide" in the history of the senses, at least in the West. In this respect, this study questions the usefulness of broadly conceived designations of a place or time as "premodern" or "modern." Not only are such terms quite problematic insofar as elements from one period often bled into the other, but, as I show, the senses generally traversed time and space in such a fugitive, roaming fashion that to frame understanding of a place and time as either premodern or modern through a history of any sense can be misleading. While I do not deny that the print revolution and its attendant developments certainly empowered vision in some important ways, I maintain that it did so quite unevenly and certainly not always at the expense of the other senses, an argument that has recently gained currency among intellectual, social, and cultural historians.[1] While I accept the premodern/modern divide as a reasonably helpful way to understand the history of the senses generally, I also use the distinction in part to show how a careful analysis of the senses begins to atrophy the distinction, and how the senses transcend the "great divide" in ways that mock a hard distinction between sensorially-indexed premodern and modern eras.

I make this argument by attending carefully to the social and cultural history of the senses. It takes the history of the everyday, the average, and the banal as seriously as it takes the history of elites, the intellect, and the exceptional, in an effort to understand the full range of meanings people attributed to the senses in the past. This book therefore intervenes at a key juncture in the evolution of writing on the history of the senses in an effort to subject prevailing narratives and frameworks to empirical test by surveying what historians from a number of fields have actually found about the senses from antiquity to modernity.[2]

The study proceeds on the understanding that the senses are historical, that they are not universal but, rather, a product of place and, especially, time, so that how people perceived and understood smell, sound, touch, taste, and sight changed historically. I agree entirely with anthropologist Constance Classen's insightful observation that "The fundamental premise underlying the concept of an 'anthropology of the senses' is that sensory perception is a cultural, as well as a physical act" and that understanding constitutes an epistemic basis of sensory history. In the West (principally Europe and North America), as Classen notes, "we are accustomed to thinking of perception as a physical act rather than a cultural act" which suggests we need to expose the senses for what they are: historically and culturally generated ways of knowing and understanding. Popular books on the senses are popular precisely because they tend to reaffirm the largely Western idea that sensing is a physical act and avoid the muddy and difficult historical treatment of the evolution of the senses.[3] And so the word "is" rarely graces the pages of this book; I do not claim that the sense of smell, taste, sight, sound, or taste "is" anything. To do so violates a fundamental point of this essay: the senses are not universal, are not transhistorical, and can only be understood in their specific social and historical contexts. The idea that a sense "is" anything does enormous violence to the central idea that senses were lots of things. Their histories cannot be understood by accepting misleading conceits concerning what a given sense supposedly means – or "is" – today, whatever that might mean.

This is an argument that I address and elaborate in the conclusion but also one that veins the body of the text.[4]

The Habit of Sensory History

While some historians refer to "the history of the senses," the history of sense perception, or, simply, "sensory history" interchangeably they often mean similar things even though there are some important distinctions to be drawn. Historians of the senses have mostly traced the evolution of a particular sense in and of itself. Some histories of hearing, for example, tend to examine how the intellectual and especially biological understanding of hearing – the ear as physiology – has evolved over time and place. Sensory history does the same but gestures towards the ecumenical, considering not only the history of a given sense but also its social and cultural construction and its role in texturing the past. It attempts to bring into dialogue historians and scholars from a variety of fields who have attended to the sensate. Sensory history obviously deals with the way that people thought about the senses, the cognitive processing of their sense perceptions, but it takes seriously the full social and cultural context of those experiences. It does not treat the senses as reducible to an intellectual history project or a history of the mind. While it certainly respects that way of understanding the senses, sensory history strives for the broadest possible framing. At its most powerful, sensory history is also explanative, allowing historians to elucidate by reference to both visual and non-visual senses something that makes little or less sense if understood simply as a scopic phenomenon. Sensory history, in short, stresses the role of the senses – including *explicit* treatments of sight and vision – in shaping peoples' experiences in the past, shows how they understood their worlds and why, is very careful not to assume that the senses are some sort of "natural" endowment, and strives not to reify the senses but, rather, locate their meaning and function in specific historical contexts.[5]

In this respect, sensory history is less a "field" of inquiry and more a habit of thinking about the past, an engrained way of exploring not just the role of sight in the past but the other senses, too. As such, sensory history is distinct from many previous historiographical and conceptual shifts mainly because it has not evolved in reaction to an established paradigm. The principle shifts in historical research in the past thirty or so years have often been generated by oppositional thinking. Thus, women's history (quite properly) evolved in part in reaction to mainstream history, largely written about and for men. So too with African American history in the United States, which responded to heavy emphasis on the history of whites (which was, by and large, proxy for general "American" history). The same may be said of micro history, which was a reaction against nationally defined narratives. More recently, interest in global history emerged out of a frustration with both local and national histories and the heuristic limitations attendant on both. Similarly, some of the recent history of consumerism sometimes seems crafted in counterpoint to the much-studied history of production. And so on.

While it is true that the history of the non-visual senses has been inspired in part by an effort to redress the heavy emphasis on seeing in much historical writing, sensory history generally is less inclined to reject vision in favor of the other senses or to define itself against a field or subject. Instead, sensory history is positioned within the coordinates of multiple fields. Thus, sensory history is more properly conceived of as a habit, a way of thinking about the past, and a way of becoming attuned to the wealth of sensory evidence embedded in any number of texts, evidence that is overwhelmingly apparent once and, ironically, *looked* for. The sensate habit is critical to sensory history not least because it pricks consciousness and questions assumptions about what to examine and how to examine it. What are usually considered historical "fields" of inquiry – diplomatic, gender, race, regional, borderlands, cultural, political, military, and so on – could all be written and researched through the habit of sensory history. Its ultimate success or failure as a habit, as an embedded way of remaining vigilant about and sensitive to the full sensory texture of the past and what the senses tell us about the nature of historical experience, will perhaps be measured in coming years less in the number of books dedicated explicitly to histories of the senses and more by the frequency with which historians generally begin to incorporate the habits of sensory history in their research and writing.

Genealogies

The recent spike in the number of studies dedicated to aspects of sensory history – as well as its increasing popular presence outside of the academy – should not obscure the habit's deeper genealogy. Although historian Robert Jütte has argued that "With the growth of interest in the body that is such a striking feature of the everyday culture of the present, the five senses are back in fashion," the historical study of the senses is not entirely indebted to histories of the body and has, in fact, been a preoccupation among some historians for a while. Certainly, scholarly interest in the history of the body, especially popular among philosophers and ethnographers in the 1980s, does help account for the rise in the interest in the sensate, but sensory history goes further than treatments of the body, which sometimes tend to flirt with the senses in an additive, even capricious, fashion rather than treating them to sustained, dedicated, historical analysis.[6]

We can identify a number of early pioneers in sensory history and, even though their remarks were often brief and embedded in a discourse usually dedicated to exploring aspects of the past that were only tangentially sensate, their tentative insights helped establish the senses as worthy of sustained historical treatment. In his 1942 work, *The Problem of Unbelief in the Sixteenth Century*, *Annales* School founder, Lucien Febvre, for example, made the bold claim that non-visual senses were more important in sixteenth-century Europe than they were in the modern era, a point that influenced Robert Mandrou's work and also helped shape Norbert Elias's thinking on the history of manners and sensibilities. Critically, Febvre advised scholars to resist the temptation to import modern understandings of what the senses may or may not mean to them into their historical research.[7]

This early work has not gone unnoticed among more recent historians of the senses. In his compelling history of religion, the American Enlightenment, and aurality, Leigh Eric Schmidt makes the intellectual debt to the *Annales* School quite explicit. Schmidt explains, for example, the relevance of Mandrou's contribution "in detailing a history of hearing loss in his inventory of the senses in early modern France." Even though Schmidt is not persuaded by some of Mandrou's claims about the apparent denigration of aurality in the modern era, he recognizes that such suggestive arguments were important for helping historians begin to think seriously about the senses and the putative victory of the visualist esthetic during and after the Enlightenment.[8]

Scholars in related disciplines have also done much to sensitize historians to the sensate, of course, and we could point to work on vision by Michel Foucault. But we should be careful not to exaggerate the importance of such work to the growing interest in sensory history, especially with regard to the non-visual senses. Foucault, after all, offered brilliant analyses but almost all of them on sight and vision as a form of surveillance. Moreover, Foucault sometimes endorsed a version of the great divide theory when he argued that observation and sight, from the seventeenth century onwards, degraded "hearsay" as well as "taste and smell" as generators of knowledge. Indeed, as David Howes and Marc Lalonde argue, the heavy emphasis Foucault placed on the ubiquity of sight, the classificatory eye, the hegemony of surveillance, and the immense popularity of his work among scholars from a variety of fields, has perhaps functioned to eclipse the enduring importance of the other, putatively lower senses of smell and taste especially, in shaping modernity, class distinctions, and notions of individualism.[9]

A breakthrough for modern historians of the senses came with the intervention of historically minded-anthropologists – most notably David Howes and Constance Classen – and with the important work of historian Alain Corbin. Beginning with his 1982 book on the history of smell – which he followed with a history of bells, sound, and a general if idiosyncratic treatment of the history of the senses (all were subsequently translated into English) – Corbin did more than any single historian to refine the insights of the early *Annales* School, elaborate them, and establish sensory history as a serious, profitable, and exciting avenue of historical inquiry.[10]

Beyond the influence of the *Annales* School, particular subfields have been more attuned to sensory history than others. European historians, especially those of medicine, have attended enthusiastically to the history of the senses, for example. As W. F. Bynum and Roy Porter noted in their introduction to the 1993 edited collection, *Medicine and the Five Senses*: "As a practical activity, medicine requires its votaries to rely on their senses to come to diagnostic judgments which in turn dictate therapeutic recommendations. As members of a learned profession, doctors are forced to ponder on the relationship between sensation and reality... As students they are taught how to use their senses and, detective-like, to interpret the clues they have picked up... The history of medicine embraces ample portions of both sense and sensibility."[11] Other historians have tended to arrive at sensory history via a number of subfields, principally those of social history, the history of religion, environmental history, the history of media and communication, urban history, the history of technology, and legal history.[12]

The cumulative effect of this scholarship generally has been significant. Just how far we have come in the past few years is apparent in George H. Roeder, Jr.'s claim that "ours is a nearly senseless profession." It was true when he wrote it; now, a decade or so later, far less so. In his pioneering article, based on a detailed search for "memorable and analytically significant smells, tastes, sights, sounds, and tactile sensations in sixteen American history textbooks" written over the past forty years, Roeder found, for example, that few textbook authors paid attention "to sensory dimensions of history" and that most sensory content (little though there was) was very much visual or of the negative sort (foul smells, pain, and noise especially, seemed most popular). By the 1980s, though, things were looking – and smelling, hearing, touching, and tasting – up. Books published after the 1970s, found Roeder, were far more likely to attend to the sensate, in part because of the growing importance of social history to the writing of American history. That much said, many of the examples offered by Roeder are less instances of an explicit, self-aware effort to get to grips with the role of the senses in shaping U.S. history and more in the service of literary, chatty flourish. Smells, noises, tastes, and touches are still passed over in many textbook narratives and all too often authors decline to explain why these senses were important or what we learn by attending to the sensory context. Roeder recognized the problem in part by showing how impoverished historians' use of sensory language was and how unprepared they were to describe sensory experience. Although great strides in textbook writing had been made since the 1970s, Roeder ended by stressing the need to "write about the senses with the same fullness and precision that we demand of ourselves when discussing politics, philosophy, or social movements." Doing so, he argued, will "enlarge our audience, our field of study, and our understanding of the past."[13]

This list by no means exhausts the genealogy of sensory history but it does give some sense of the evolution of sensory history and, moreover, suggests how relatively underdeveloped the subject matter and habit remains. Keep in mind the scores of books published annually on, say, the American Civil War and it becomes clear that sensory history is still, despite a great deal of very recent work, very much in its infancy.

The Great Divide

Arguably, the most influential framework shaping how historians have examined the senses is by Marshall McLuhan and Walter Ong, the principal architects of orality theory or the "great divide" theory, as it is sometimes called.

David Howes, in a brilliant essay summarizing the various incarnations of "great divide" theories, says this of McLuhan's work: "controversially, McLuhan sought to explain all of human history, as well as the differences in social organization between the West and the 'tribal' societies of Africa and the Orient, in terms of transformations in the 'ratio of the senses' brought on by changes in the technology of communications." In *The Gutenberg Galaxy: The Making of Typographic Man* (1962) and *Understanding Media: The Extensions of Man* (1965), McLuhan offered a series of sophisticated arguments about language, technology, and the relationship among the various senses – but especially between sight and hearing – in a number of societies and argued that cultures and the histories that shape them are best conceived of as differential extensions of the senses.[14]

The argument maintains that following the invention of movable type in the sixteenth century and under the ensuing influence of an eye-centered Renaissance and Enlightenment, vision came to dominate Western thinking, serving as authenticator of truth, courier of reason, and custodian of the intellect, while the senses of taste, touch, and smell, especially, were essentially sidelined. More specifically, according to McLuhan, the basic sensory arrangements unfolded along four stages: oral–aural, chirographic (essentially, hand-written), typographic, and electronic. In oral–aural societies, speech constituted the basis of communication and, as such, shaped the nature of collective thought and behavior, arranging sensory ratios in a particular way. Here, given the preeminence of speech, hearing figures prominently as does tactility and olfaction (people grouped together to communicate and touches and smells were part of that "synesthetic" communicative medium). In McLuhan's reckoning, all preliterate, pre-print societies, including what he calls the "tribal" societies of Africa, manifested the same ear-dominated but essentially synesthetic sensorium. The chirographic stage sees the unraveling of this sensory unity because it replaces orality-aurality with visuality. The phonetic alphabet is critical in this disassociation, argues McLuhan: only it "has the power to translate man from the tribal to the civilized sphere, to give him an eye for an ear." To be sure, the triumph of the eye over the other senses was still uncertain during this stage. "Manuscript culture," says McLuhan, "is intensely audile-tactile compared to print culture; and that means that detached habits of observation are quite uncongenial to manuscript cultures, whether ancient Egyptian, Greek, or Chinese. In place of cool visual detachment the manuscript world puts empathy and participation of all the senses." Consider, for example, what was involved in reading: "in the Middle Ages, as in antiquity, they read usually, not as today, principally with their eyes, but with the lips, pronouncing what they saw, and with the ears, listening to the words pronounced, hearing what is called the 'voices of the pages.'"[15]

For McLuhan, it was the printing press that ushered in Guttenberg's sensory galaxy, a world in which seeing became preeminent and the importance of the other senses dulled and lessened. Texts became standardized (eliminating the vagaries of handwriting), reproducible on a large scale, and came to be apprehended in purely visual form. As such, the print revolution was also responsible for braiding sight and logic, seeing and reason, vision and objectivity. McLuhan and Walter Ong were in close agreement on this fundamental issue and quoted one another approvingly. Unlike sound and speech which, they claimed, penetrated and surrounded listeners (often quite emotionally), sight – so empowered by print – objectified what was seen, giving the viewer perspective, distance, balance, coolness, detachment, and a growing sense of self. It was this visual hegemony that characterized, for McLuhan, Western society from the Renaissance until fairly late in the twentieth century as well as marking the separation of Western society form "tribal," oral–aural societies, which took much longer to embrace written and print technologies. For McLuhan, the final stage, the electronic age, reunited the senses. The eye no longer reigned supreme. Television and radio, for example, resurrected aurality, and helped Western youth appreciate the desirability of tactility.[16]

The great divide model was imaginative, thought-provoking, erudite, and sweeping and offered a generation of thinkers and scholars of media and history and technological and social change a productive way to think about the history of the senses. But these strengths should not distract us from it difficulties. Part of the problem in evaluating the ongoing relevance and helpfulness of work by McLuhan, Ong, and others is that they themselves often refined their positions, thus making it difficult to talk authoritatively of, say, Ong's "position." Critically, as Howes has argued, when attending to Ong's work especially, historians are better served distinguishing between his early and later work, relying more on the historically informed 1967 book, *The Presence of the Word*, and taking less seriously the teleology of his later work – as outlined in *Orality and Literacy* (1982) – which champions a more radical and binary "great divide" theory.[17]

In *The Presence of the Word*, Ong stressed the interdependency of the senses and how their ranking and use changed over time. The book is full of talk about the enduring relevance of, for example, tactility long after the advent of writing and print, how touch and sight combined even as visuality became preeminent. Ong also found the senses of taste and hearing trumping vision in some quarters during the eighteenth century – the supposed century of visualism. Ong sometimes slipped toward a dichotomous model in *The Presence of the Word*, even as he spoke in terms of sensory ratio shifts. For example, he claimed, "In general, before the invention of script man is more oral–aural than afterward," and, "Writing, most particularly the alphabet," but also the advent of print and perspectival painting in the fifteenth century, combined to shift "the balance of the senses away from the aural to the visual." But, for the most part, Ong avoided postulating a stubbornly binary model by noting how different media – and their sensory ratios – "do not abolish one another but overlie one another." Therein is Ong's theoretical flexibility, a position from which he retreats in his later work which while acknowledging the often slow, piecemeal, and stuttered emergence of visualism, nonetheless offers a framework stressing discontinuity. "[T]he shift from oral to written speech," he tells us in *Orality and Literacy*, "is essentially a shift from sound to visual space." His position here retains less of the flux and overlap of his previous formulation. For Howes, Ong's position in *Orality and Literacy*, with its "fundamental duality of sense experience – ear/eye, oral literate" is an unfortunate declension from the more helpful, earlier formulation emphasizing "the idea of shifts in the 'ratio or balances of the senses,'" a model containing "a great wealth of potential applications."[18]

Sensory history remains deeply indebted to the pioneering work of McLuhan, Ong, and others. Whatever its collective shortcoming – which I'll outline shortly – their work established the importance of the senses to understanding the past and made critical connections between technology, the relationships among the senses, and helped us understand the historical importance of the print revolution.[19]

Beyond the Great Divide

For all its brilliance, there is, from an historian's perspective in particular, a great deal that is quite disconcerting about the great divide or orality theory. McLuhan's *Gutenberg Galaxy* especially offers a hermeneutic laced with zero-sum binaries, with eyes and ears frequently portrayed as mutually exclusive. Moreover, some of his claims are so broad and sweeping as to have very little historical worth. "The Chinese," McLuhan tells us at one point, "are tribal, people of the ear," an observation that begs rather than answers questions.[20]

Yet the binary quality of the great divide theory itself has proven attractive to some scholars, perhaps because it seemingly allows for broad, rhetorically satisfying statements about historical change and group values. In his otherwise excellent treatment of the legal history of the senses, Bernard Hibbitts says that the invention of the printing press, the universalization of literacy, and the cultural hegemony of literate groups created a new world order, a sensory holocaust in which "spoken rhetoric was denigrated. Gestures were demeaned... Smells and tastes were stricken from the accepted vocabulary of literary expression." Even though Hibbitts later – and more reliably – talks convincingly about how print inaugurated merely a shift in sensory ratios the appeal of a binary great divide theory can distract even very fine minds and induce reckless analysis.[21]

There is irony here. Some scholars cleave to the great divide theory, and McLuhan's powerful articulation of it especially, because of its historical content and apparent explanative power. Historical pivots and identifiable turning points can seem satisfying in and of themselves. Yet McLuhan was not an especially good historian. His evidence was largely literary – hardly surprising given that he earned his doctorate in English literature – and often lacked detail and a sense of context. Moreover, scholars such as Hibbitts tend to have imported the least helpful aspects of McLuhan's work into their thinking and left his best insights languishing and underdeveloped. For example, McLuhan was careful to talk about the print revolution initiating a shift in sensory ratios, so that sight simply became more important than the other senses under modernity. This, in itself, is a very valuable insight, and allows us to think in terms of how the senses are combined in a given society, how they work together, and advances the notion of intersensorality and how the senses articulated, an idea only now being taken seriously by historians. That some scholars have been more intrigued by McLuhan's less subtle great divide theory is unfortunate because this aspect of McLuhan's argument was over-theorized, under-researched, and took on an absolute quality, one that can leave readers with the impression that preliterate societies are exclusively oral-aural and emotional and that literate societies are exclusively visual and rational. Such an association not only fails to stand up to scrutiny but the idea is essentially ahistorical. Senses and their meaning are not universal but, rather, hostage to time and place and, as such, any claim that sight is wholly rational or that the other senses are unintellectual has to be tested empirically, not simply claimed theoretically.

A few anthropologists have been critical of aspects of McLuhan's work specifically and the great divide and orality theory generally. David Howes, for example, has rightly wondered whether McLuhan overemphasized the tension between eye and ear and downplayed the others senses. "There should be more to the notion of 'sensory ratio' than meets the eye or reverberates in the ear," writes Howes. Similarly, Constance Classen suggests how easy it is to overstate the triumph of visualism. "The sensory world of Renaissance Europe, while affected by the shifting sensory values of the modern age, was grounded in traditional practices and beliefs retained from the ancient and medieval periods," she argues, elaborating: "Thus while sight was customarily considered the highest of the senses, it was still insufficient to convey a complete 'picture' of the world." The other senses, often in tandem, were critical for communicating religious, social, and cultural information. Classen warns against treating language, spoken and written, as excessively visual and aural-oral. Writing, she points out, was tactile and visual while speech was often olfactory as well as oral.[22]

Historian of religion, Leigh Eric Schmidt, also criticizes Ong and McLuhan, finding both too binary in their formulations. For Schmidt, sound – especially in the context of religious hearing during the American Enlightenment of the late eighteenth and early nineteenth centuries – was inextricable to vision and he refuses to posit "hard-and-fast oppositions," preferring instead to examine the historical unfolding of the sensory relationship between sound and vision. Although this is, in fact, similar to some of what Ong (at least in *The Presence of the Word*) and McLuhan advocated, Schmidt prefers, quite understandably, to frame his work beyond the great divide framework, appealing instead to a model stressing historically situated "multisensory complexity." As Schmidt rightly remarks: "The modern sensorium remains more intricate and uneven, its perceptual disciplines and experiential modes more diffuse and heterogeneous, than the discourses of Western visuality and ocularcentrism allow."[23]

Refreshing the Ratios: Re(envisioning) the Past

One reason why the great divide theory continues to cast a long shadow over a good deal of writing on the history of the senses is because some of that history and historiography is a product of a particular style of intellectual history, a form of historical inquiry and writing that tends to find sympathy with the sort of project and argument offered by McLuhan and Ong. No small amount of historical writing on the history of the senses has been performed by intellectual historians who have traced the way senses and their meanings have preoccupied great thinkers, especially in the Western cannon. The dividends of this emphasis are undeniable: we know what a range of thinkers thought about the senses, especially from the seventeenth century on in Western history. But we should be careful not to allow intellectual discourses on the senses to be our sole guide. Many – although, as I'll suggest, by no means all – seventeenth- and eighteenth-century intellectuals were inclined to see events through Enlightenment eyes and they tended to privilege sight even as they discussed in meaningful fashion the function of the other senses. In this regard, McLuhan came to the conclusions he did in part because he relied on a certain kind of evidence from intellectuals to tell his story.

Take, for example, Robert Jütte's otherwise excellent 2005 study, *History of the Senses*. Jütte's epistemology tends to work within the coordinates of the great divide theory. He relies heavily on an intellectual history of the senses which, in turn, allows him to stress how the revolution in print and the imperatives of the Enlightenment inaugurated the "reign of the eye and the sense of vision." A more flexible theoretical framework, one less indebted to the great divide or orality theory, one more invested in the social and cultural history of the senses would have helped Jütte explain more fully the historical significance of the continued relevance of non-visual senses under modernity.[24]

A fuller engagement with social and cultural history and a sincere attempt to bring that work into dialogue with the often very thoughtful work of intellectual historians of the senses suggests that non-visual senses remained central to the elaboration of modernity in many of its forms and configurations even as vision rose in importance. Vision's power did not devalue the other senses in an experiential sense as much as a strict interpretation and application of the great divide model suggests. A social and cultural history of the senses, then, tends to show that non-visual ways of understanding the world retained their importance even after the invention of print – which was a more protracted affair than either McLuhan or Ong suggest – and the flourishing of Enlightenment ideas. While it is certainly the case that intellectual histories of the senses can grant us access to core values, historians have to be very careful about which voices and which values they listen to in the process of uncovering the past. Listen to intellectual voices, to thinkers concerned with the philosophical, abstract functioning of the senses, and one particular, often vision-centered version of Western history emerges; listen to voices recovered most often by social and cultural history, and a more balanced, if more complicated, picture emerges. Some thinkers, of course, understood the social importance of the senses (Karl Marx comes to mind especially), some wrote eloquently on the importance of understanding experience as located sensorially, and some intellectual discourse (notably in twentieth-century France) developed radically antiocular critiques, very likely because their society and culture was so increasingly spectacular and visualist. But many intellectuals, as Jütte's fine book shows, while noting the existence of the other, non-visual senses, tended to reaffirm the supremacy of vision and the specific set of power relations embedded in that way of seeing the world. As Alain Corbin has argued, we must stress the primacy of context if we are to avoid becoming hostage to the rhetorical sensory hierarchy sponsored by a given class of a particular place and time. Rather, he argues, we must understand the actual ways in which people understood the senses, their relation, and their social meaning, and to do that demands that we listen to multiple voices from multiple contexts and discourses.[25]

Corbin further explains how sight was constructed as antithetical to the so-called proximate senses to mirror critical class distinctions in late eighteenth- and nineteenth-century France. The delicate, refined, elite spectator viewed with studied gaze the violent mob and massacres of late eighteenth-century France from a distance, developing a visual, "spectatorial" attitude for both understanding and assigning the meaning of mob behavior. Seeing massacre was enough to instill in the spectator "horror" and repulsion. Conversely, according to Corbin, the member of the mob who was actively engaged in the violence and murder, the one "who receives its sounds and smells," who mediates the experience and understanding of the event through "the senses of proximity," of touch and smell especially, constituted a sensorially delimited class, one separate from the visually inclined elite spectator. But Corbin is far too clever an historian to be lured here. Here, "surreptitiously, we are falling into the trap which consists, for the historian, of confusing the reality of the employment of the senses and the picture of this employment decreed by observers." In other words, some evidence concerning the primacy of vision comes from sources that are historically suspect because they were promoted by elites for elites. Frequently, the descriptions we have of the use of the senses were established by – and left by – elites, which likely reflect their preferred understanding of reality, but not reality in its full, multivalent, contingent texture. For us to assume that vision was triumphant is also to assume the accuracy and innocence of the discourse that describes it. Instead, what we need is more and better evidence to see to what extent elites quietly engaged the proximate senses and where French peasants and workers were more visual than elite rhetoric would suggest.[26]

We now possess enough studies by social and cultural historians on the history of the senses to critically reexamine the great divide theory and standard claims about the emerging hegemony of the eye. These studies can, and should, be read alongside and in dialogue with – and not in opposition to – important work by a number of intellectual historians who have themselves done much to dilute the association between modernity and the eye. Had McLuhan had ready access to the number and range of social and cultural histories of the senses and the sort of intellectual history that interrogates the reliability of the eye, he would likely have qualified some of his more emphatic statements about the triumph of vision.[27]

I am not the first to make the claim that social history broadens and revises our understanding of sensory history in fundamental ways. A good deal of my analysis in this book is premised on the foundational insight offered by Constance Classen, namely: "Even without a Marxist history of the senses, Marxist theory has certainly influenced sensory historians and cultural historians in general to undertake a history 'from below,' from the perspective of workers and peasants as well as the ruling classes, and to take account of the role of class interests in promulgating social and sensory ideologies." Classen further explains that a social history of the senses "invites an exploration into the culture of the senses because of the traditional association in the West of the 'lower' classes with the body and sensuality" while being careful not to accept historical conceits concerning the putative sensuality of the poor.[28]

Similarly, Alan Hunt, in his fascinating examination of the history of sumptuary law, found the same messiness and contingency that I find for sensory history not least because he relied not just on elite sources but also a reading of a broadly constituted social history. Conventional wisdom regarding sumptuary law was, like histories of the senses, pivoted very much on the premodern/modern historical divide. Traditional work was resolutely teleological and Whiggish, depicting sumptuary law as premodern, typical of aristocratic and absolutist quirks, their decline best explained by the emergence of the idea of private rights and democracy. But Hunt's attention to social history found that sumptuary law was deeply implicated in the emergence of modernity and helped shape not only social class but also influenced gender ideals.[29]

My position in this book is to suspend the unhelpful binary aspects of Ong's and McLuhan's work and build on their insights concerning intersensorality under modernity. This, it seems to me, is very much in keeping with Corbin's position and allows us to investigate the relative strength of vision before and after the print revolution in relation to the other senses without necessarily accepting the formulation positing vision as the preeminent sense of the modern era. In other words, while I wish to take full note of the undeniable importance of the ocular to modernity, empowered as it was by the developments noted by Ong and McLuhan, I do not wish to assume that all of the other senses were wholly subordinate or that, conversely, the premodern era downplayed the importance of sight in favor of the non-visual senses. We now possess enough work on the history of the senses over time and place – and not just for the West – to profitably subject theoretical statements about the nature of the great divide and sensory shifts to some empirical test.[30]

To frame understanding of the history of the senses along the unstable and withered axes of the great divide theory runs the risk of using the senses to "other" the very people of the past we seek to understand and, in fact, were frequently the victims of othering, courtesy of the aggressive deployment of sensory stereotypes, by their more powerful contemporaries. Without careful and precise contextualization and historicization that pays attention to the senses as relative cultural constructs, we are in danger of reinscribing an historical conceit that makes the past simply more sensual just because it was the past. As Mark Jenner has perceptively remarked with regard to the historical study of smell: to describe the past as smellier is not only to avoid engagement with what contemporaries defined as smell but, more seriously and inextricably, reinscribes "the notion that the remote past was marked by squalor and stench, and modernity by a *nostalgie de la merde*." Simple claims that the distant past was a time and place where odors were stronger simply "construct[s] a narrative of progress and deodorization," a claim that needs testing rather than mere declaration. Olfaction was no more a "natural" sense in the sixteenth century than in the twentieth and to suggest otherwise dehistoricizes the senses and simply restates the claims of some eighteenth- and nineteenth-century European reformers who claimed that civilization had tamed stench. Some of these claims might be true, of course, but, as Jenner suggests, we need to be very careful about repeating them in the absence of evidence that takes account of change over time and space. Only with that sort of context-sensitive historical inquiry can we profitably begin to ask serious questions about the relationship between the rise of print culture, ideas concerning perspective, the Enlightenment, vision, and sight's relationship to the other senses and to broadly construed premodern and modern societies.[31]

In other words, the evidence we have from social and cultural historians – as well as from some intellectual histories – regarding the senses for both modern and premodern periods suggests that we must be careful not to overstate the extent of the elevation of the eye following the print revolution and the Enlightenment, nor to understate the importance of vision to so-called premodern societies. We should also try to understand that the project of modernity was necessarily indebted to the proximate senses as much as it was to vision. Modernity – the categorization of races, industrialization, the creation of elites and working classes, the invention of gender roles, the project of imperialism, the creation of multiple others – could not be effected by sight alone. It is only through a history that attends as much to the social experience and development of the senses as it does to class and gender specific, usually elite, intellectual constructions and discourses, that we can make sense of making sense.[32]

Because this book functions principally as a primer and as an introduction to work on the topic, it is structured around showing how historians have used and understood each sense. Although structurally the book replicates the traditional sensory hierarchy – beginning with sight, the supposedly most noble sense, and ending with touch, often described as the least intellectual of the senses – it does not reinscribe or empower that hierarchy. Neither does it seek, as the Conclusion makes clear, to arrange the supposedly proximate senses of smell, taste, and touch against those of sight or hearing. Rather, and as will become clear, the book's structure reflects the nature and amount of historical work done on each sense and functions simply to replicate the way that most scholars have understood the arrangement of the senses historically. That much said, I have been careful to show in each chapter how the senses sometimes functioned together; how, for example, smell and taste frequently operated in conjunction at a given moment in time for a particular group, even though the chapter concerned details, principally, the history and historiography of olfaction. My aim is not to invert standard sensory hierarchies or to reaffirm them. Rather, it is to complicate them and that can only be done with any real profit by attending to the history of the senses in a fully historicized fashion over many places and arcing over a long period of time.

1

Seeing

Look Here: Seeing the Light

Taking the history of the senses seriously – and not simply invoking them as a literary device to spice narrative – is challenging, not least because ways of "viewing" the past are deeply embedded in the writing and understanding of history generally. According to a number of visual studies scholars, seeing has long occupied something of a hegemonic position in Western culture "due to the association of sight with both scientific rationalism and capitalist display and to the expansion of the visual field by means of technologies of observation and reproduction – from the telescope to the television." Thus, not only have we tended to study seeing and vision more than the other senses (the historiography of vision is much deeper than that of the other senses combined), not only have we tended to ignore the so-called "lower" senses, but in both cases, we have done so through a largely unconscious ocularcentrist or retinalphilic "lens" which, courtesy of Renaissance, scientific, and Enlightenment developments, has informed our drive for scholarly "perspective," our search for "focus," and other visual ways of understanding the past that quietly tether rational "truth" to a stable, cool, authenticating eye. And despite recent efforts to restore the other senses to the study of the past, vision still guides a good deal of scholarly and historical work. "Even critiques of the dominance of sight," argues David Howes, "tend to remain within the realm of vision and rarely consider what alternatives to hypervisuality might lie within other sensory domains, or emerge from combining the senses in new ratios."[1]

This is not to understate the importance of some marvelous work on the history of vision and seeing, on visual culture generally; nor is it to call for a moratorium on work detailing the history of vision. The importance of sensory history lies not in segregating the senses but, rather, in exploring their interplay and any effort to do so without attending to the history of sight is obviously doomed. Moreover, art historians and intellectual histories of sight in particular have enabled us to identify key shifts in the history of seeing and help explain ways in which visuality became so powerful in the West. They detail the rise of print culture, the advent of scientific and technological instruments that empowered the eye, and outline Enlightenment quests for visualist perspective and balance. But while some intellectual histories of vision have been helpful in explicitly identifying seeing as one sense among many, a few also tend to tout the preeminence of sight. Thus, while Martin Jay's pioneering work traces not only the visualist impulses in print, photography, the experience of time, and in a slew of other venues, and notes the emergence of an anti-ocular critique associated with key French writers and intellectuals (Derrida, Barthes, Sartre, Merleau-Ponty, Lacan, among others), he sometimes ends up reiterating the centrality of sight.[2] As Steven Connor explains, sight is tenacious, even when interrogated. Connor outlines why, for example, the modern self – "the epistemized self which takes itself as an object of self-knowledge" – is typically (if inaccurately) understood in terms of visuality. Seeing, shows Connor, has been the principal category by which the modern self has been understood to frame the world and separate it as an object of knowledge, understanding, and manipulation.[3] Connor illustrates this tendency in Jay's work. Although Jay shows how the idea of vision has been questioned even as the ocular became consolidated, Connor points out that Jay's investigation of seeing ironically reinstates the importance of the eye, often at the expense of the other senses and their role in shaping notions of the self. In "the many examples of antiocularcentrism arrayed by Martin Jay," offers Connor, "the suspicion of sight often takes the more abstract form of an intensified scrutiny of vision, a scrutiny which amounts to a kind of vision raised to a higher power."[4]

More generally, it is fair to say that a good deal of scholarly indifference to the non-visual senses is largely unwitting, a product of (ocular) habit, not design. Most historians have not been actively hostile to attending to the sensate; rather, they have simply been hostage to seeing history through eyes rather than trying to understand the olfactory, tactile, auditory, or gustatory aspects of the past. In a way, of course, historians have always "done" sensory history, simply because they have relied heavily on the sense of sight to frame the past. Constance Classen and David Howes have recently – and rightly – remarked that "Of course, much has been written about the 'complexities' of visual culture in modernity, and much, no doubt, remains to be written. Yet our academic focus on vision must not be allowed to defer indefinitely the investigation of the social life of non-visual sensory phenomena."[5]

More than that, though, the stress on seeing serves in some ways to reinscribe the value of the eye in the very writing of history and, for our understanding of the modern, post-Enlightenment period especially, reaffirms, rather than interrogates, prevailing frameworks stressing the victory of the rational eye under modernity. Historical work on the history of sight – for both the pre- and post-Enlightenment eras – has often echoed the deeply ingrained association between the eye and the intellect. While we know a great deal about the intellectual history of seeing, we are now beginning to get a better idea of the social and cultural history of vision, how ideas about seeing were influenced by, for example, constructions of gender and race. This chapter, while necessarily mindful of the important work by intellectual historians on seeing and the work of visual studies scholars generally pays careful attention to the way social and cultural historians have investigated the history of visuality. Combined, the work of some intellectual historians and offerings by some social and cultural historians of the senses, as well as key works by students of philosophy and literature, suggests that the print revolution and the Enlightenment did not empower vision as much as is sometimes assumed.

The Eyes Have It: Seeing and Believing in the Modern West

We should not, of course, jettison some of the fundamental insights of the great divide theory when it comes to understanding the importance of sight. A good deal of evidence supports the larger argument that the print revolution and the Enlightenment did, in fact, elevate the eye.

The great divide theory has earned endorsements from a variety of talented thinkers and historians. Donald Lowe, for example, in his important study, *History of Bourgeois Perception*, identifies the relationship between modernity and sight by tracing the emergence of a "new perceptual field, constituted by typographic culture" and "the primacy of sight" that triumphed at the expense of non-visual senses. Some philosophical treatments have also stressed how very embedded vision is to modernity. According to David Michael Levin, "our Western culture has been dominated by an ocularcentric paradigm, a vision-generated, vision-centered interpretation of knowledge, truth, and reality." Vision's tendency to fix, reify, and totalize, he maintains, has given rise to an "ocularcentric metaphysics of presence" one that, in his opinion, needs to be challenged. Legal scholar, Bernard Hibbitts, also makes a case for the sensory impact of the invention of writing and script. As he explains: "One of the greatest strengths of writing as a medium is its technological capacity physically to separate the sender of a message from its recipient... Writing thus discourages simultaneous reliance on speech, gesture, touch, and savor."[6]

Some scholars have also found it helpful to read the history of acoustemology and hearing within the coordinates of the larger great divide theory. R. Murray Schafer, for example, arguably the doyen of soundscape studies, maintains that "In the West the ear gave way to the eye as the most important gatherer of information about the time of the Renaissance, with the development of the printing press and perspective painting." Schafer is clearly persuaded by the arguments concerning the shift in the ratio of the senses – and our own apparent return to the ear – offered by McLuhan.[7] Most recently, Richard Rath's important study of soundways in colonial America offers a qualified but sympathetic endorsement of the great divide theory. Although, as Rath rightly remarks, "Most historians ... take no account of the perceptual shift" that preoccupies Ong and McLuhan, those that do tend to take seriously Ong's early work and McLuhan's more subtle formulations concerning the ratio of the senses. Rath, for example, argues that "Sound was not overcome by vision in eighteenth-century America. It is fruitless to say sound is more important than vision or vice versa. Both are necessary components of any culture's perceptual field." Although Rath clearly understands that the rise of vision only lessened the importance of sound and did not eclipse it entirely, he nevertheless sees vision indexed tightly to modernity and a consequence of print and literacy. Although Rath does not consider aurality/orality necessarily in tension with literacy – he considers belief in the tension itself a modern convention and one hardly recognizable to the people he studies – he nevertheless agrees with McLuhan's essential insight, insisting, "early Americans sensed the world more through their ears than we do today." Rath maintains that as "literacy and printed matter came closer to saturating North Americans' minds ... attention was drawn away from the realm of sound and speech in order to give more to the visible world."[8]

The importance of sight to the modern era, at least in the West, is beyond doubt not least because lots of other forces in addition to the invention of print served to empower vision. The "hyper-visual esthetic" of modernity identified by David Howes is traceable to the invention and subsequent dissemination of linear visual perspective, most often associated with Leon Battista Alberti (1404–1472), the early Renaissance Italian architect and artist. Alberti in effect placed a grid over space and fixed the eye, training it to "see" in a perspectival, balanced, and "rational" manner. This way of seeing helped establish a notion of "self," a spectator viewing the world, supposedly detached and observing. Alberti's work – and the associated developments of the Renaissance – were critical for disciplining the sensorium. As Howes puts it, Alberti's grid "screens out all the smells and sounds, tastes and textures, of the artist's environment. It 'steps up' the natural power of the eye to survey things from afar, while at the same time de-emphasizing the other senses as ways of knowing and communicating." The modern, Western eye became, in Joy Parr's telling description, at once "cold, clean, and objective," thoroughly Cartesian and geometric. It offered the illusion of order but because it went no further than the surface, it did not infuse or "feel", lost "touch with other sensuous resonances and, by oversight, marginalize[d] them." Moreover, sight, operating "at a distance and with some power over the viewed, inferentially and contingently, is masculine." Vision also became increasingly distanced from the other senses in the eighteenth and nineteenth centuries as it became handmaiden to rationalist science. Knowledge was gained through the gaze of the scientist and verified through the eye. In fact, science seemed to champion sight as the *sine qua non* of truth independently of political and economic systems. Capitalist or communist, vision and science were bedfellows. In the Soviet Union in the 1940s, for example, hearing was considered "inferior to seeing." "This truth was constantly hammered into our heads by our teacher of physics" recalled one Russian.[9]

Vision was bolstered by myriad developments and their sheer variety and social and cultural depth helps explain why the eye became so revered as an important source of truth and knowledge. Even certain art forms – beyond the obvious perspectival painting – also inscribed heavy visualism. Ballet, rooted in sixteenth- and seventeenth-century European courts, was part of political and social spectacle from the beginning. Bodily movement, precision, flow, control were all captured in ballet and constituted "visible signs of moral states, political power, political resistance, and divine association." Beyond its political implications, ballet was lodged firmly in the eye: mirrors were critical to bodily training, performers went to lengths to minimize the sounds of their steps and breathing, bestowing at once a silent and hyper-visual quality on the performance, and performers aimed to look similar. Even when other senses came into play (the touch was intrinsic to the *pas de deux*), how the touch looked to a spectator guided the choreography. It was this hypervisualism that led to the association between ballet, bodily discipline, social control, and elite interest. Working classes, by contrast, preferred noisy clog dances, thoroughly loud and vibrating, resolutely energetic, body parts flailing, at least to elite ways of looking and hearing.[10]

By the mid-nineteenth century, many Europeans certainly considered sight the preeminent esthetic sense. In England, the shift from a multi-sensorial to a largely visual appreciation of art occurred within a fairly delimited fifty-year period, some time between the 1780s and 1840s. In the 1780s, museum visitors were accustomed to, for example, touching artifacts, feeling their texture and weight and thereby gauging something about the past society that produced them. But by 1844 the writer Anna Jameson could remark, "we can all remember the loiterers and loungers ... people who, instead of moving among the wonders and beauties ... with reverence and gratitude, strutted about as if they had a right to be there; talking, flirting; touching the ornaments – and even the pictures!" Of course, Jameson was articulating a class conceit in part and using sensory esthetics to construct otherness – she suggests that only the more plebeian touched art – but even in that class construction we see how sight had become, for elites at least, the sense of judgment and taste. Touching was now uncivilized and damaging; only sight was safe, distanced, and true.[11]

Sight, certainly during and after the seventeenth century, also became increasingly important to the study and practice of Western medicine. Physicians emphasized the importance and power of visual observation and stressed the importance of signs in outward appearance, the patient's facial expressions, skin tone, color of blood and urine, and any number of visual clues. This was followed by the actual visual penetration of the body by sight in the form of the autopsy which, in turn, intensified with the ability to photograph the patient's body, and, ultimately, penetrate it with X-rays and microscopes.[12]

Even trends and developments frequently in tension served to elevate the eye and downplay the other senses. For example, both the Protestant Reformation and emerging scientific paradigms, while often fraught on key religious and ontological matters, nevertheless promoted the value of sight. The Protestant Reformation, with its emphasis on the written word and admonitions against sensualism, was certainly important in shifting sensory ratios. "The church," as Constance Classen has explained, "according to the Reformation ideal, was a place of sensory simplicity, purified of incense" and sensualism generally. And as the print revolution took hold, producing more and more books, "literate Europeans relied less on such non-visual means of accessing the divine as smelling odors of sanctity and tasting the body and blood of Christ and relied more on reading the Word of God." Science also became increasingly visual, relying on observable events and touting the supremacy of quantification as a means to access truth. The invention and dissemination of visual technologies that extended the reach of the eye – such as telescopes, glasses, and microscopes – further elevated seeing. Ironically, then, religion and science ended up agreeing on the supremacy of vision. For both, seeing became associated with believing and truth while the other senses became associated with gut, feeling, intuition, and non-verifiable, subjective emotions.[13]

Other aspects of modernity functioned similarly. Urbanization and the reconfiguration of space generally owed much to the eye and, in turn, further strengthened sight. In the eighteenth and nineteenth centuries, in place of the dark, tight, crowded streets of the medieval period – environments also associated with dingy smells, proximate touches, and transgressive noises – emerged newly designed urban spaces with broad avenues, geometric thoroughfares, and generally bright – and, increasingly lighted – environments. Public space became increasingly subject to visual surveillance, courtesy of prisons, schools, police forces, and street lighting. The eye seemingly reigned and was the custodian of state-defined safety and modernity, imposing reason on society at large.[14]

The eye also served to generate and shape particular power relations, especially in Europe during the eighteenth and nineteenth centuries, as the pioneering work of Michel Foucault shows. Modern states relied less on the use of spectacle – such as public execution – and more on less obvious, but nonetheless sight-indebted, mechanisms of surveillance; ways of normalizing behavior in order to generate and then perpetuate relations of dominance and subordination. For Foucault, the modern state actively managed the definition, ownership, and circulation of knowledge to produce obedient citizens who acted in the interest of the state not because they were obviously coerced – as in totalitarian societies – but because they accepted social norms of cooperation. For Foucault, the key to the process of acceptance lay in how citizens came to internalize a sort of managerial gaze – the eye of the state. Nowhere was this more obvious than in the Panopticon, a visually sophisticated way to inspire discipline among English prison inmates at the end of the eighteenth century. Designed by legal theorist and Utilitarian philosopher, Jeremy Bentham, the "all-seeing" Panopticon placed the inspector in the center of the structure, a position from which he could monitor inmate behavior. Foucault explained: "The Panopticon is a machine for dissociating the see/being seen dyad: in the peripheric ring, one is totally seen, without ever seeing; in the central tower, one sees everything without ever being seen." For Foucault, the power of the Panopticon lay less in the fact that prisoners were observed at all times and rather in the fact that they never really knew if and when they were being surveyed. "Bentham laid down the principle that power should be visible and unverifiable," argued Foucault, elaborating: "Visible: the inmate will constantly have before his eyes the tall outline of the central tower from which he is spied upon. Unverifiable: the inmate must never know whether he is being looked at at any one moment; but he must be sure that he may always be so." The Panopticon was an example of a wider culture of surveillance (evidenced in schools, hospitals, and empowered by the advent of photography), one dedicated to controlling bodies and one rooted in visuality (and assumptions about surveillance, being seen, and the nature of looking). Perhaps more than any other modern theorist, Foucault has often been interpreted as placing sight at the center of modern elaborations of knowledge and power.[15]

Students of the history of night and lighting technologies have, albeit implicitly, also done much to sustain this association of modernity with vision. Such work has shown that prior to the eighteenth century, most cities anywhere had little or no public street lighting. Individuals traveled at night in urban areas using torches or lanterns. Urbanization and industrialization in the nineteenth century especially increased the demand for street lights, allowing city dwellers to extend time into artificially illuminated evening and night hours. Gas and, later, electric street lighting also became cheaper and was understood not only as a way to increase economic productivity but also to secure the night against crime. Street lights were also an affordable way for a city to lay claim to modernity. They were cheaper than other infrastructural initiatives that tended to the other senses – sewer works to protect the nose, for example, were very costly endeavors – and nineteenth-century municipal authorities from Europe to South America publicly described their cities as "modern" on the basis of street lighting and their mastery of the dark.[16]

Critically, these developments gave rise to a sense of individualism – the idea of a self, demarcated, and with boundaries – which, in turn, helped establish and elaborate gender and class distinctions.

Michel de Montaigne, for example, wrote in the sixteenth century that men understood themselves on the basis of their outward and verifiable appearance whereas women and ordinary people tended to rely on a subjective and, hence, more emotional, plastic, and less visual understanding of selfhood. Such elite male thinking placed the individual at center stage in society, served to contain sensate interaction, and gave rise to the modern expression "look but don't touch." The idea of the individual self required that "people had to take greater care not to transgress the sensory space of others with untoward odors, noises, or touches." In urban areas in particular, they could not touch, taste, or smell strangers – they could only look at them. In these, and myriad other ways, the sense of self was enriched and seeing stood at the center of the process.[17]

Re-Visionist Perspectives I

To what extent did the rise of seeing and vision really discount or deflate the authority of the other senses? McLuhan's treatment – and those persuaded by his analysis – often implicitly suggest that non-visual senses lost a great deal of their meaning and value as a result of the print revolution and associated developments. The shift in the ratio, in other words, seems quite radical. Social and cultural histories of the senses, however, suggest that we should be careful to understand the importance of the emergence of sight for the reasons McLuhan suggested but not to exaggerate its significance under modernity, nor to downplay its importance in the premodern era, and not to dismiss the importance of the other senses in helping inform modernity. The other senses were not marginalized because vision triumphed. On the contrary, modernity reenergized them and was, in turn, informed by them, sometimes at the expense of seeing. In fact, we can extend Walter Ong's astute analysis that precisely because sight was sometimes understood to reveal "only surfaces" because it could "never get to an interior as an interior," modernity's preoccupation with authenticity and essence necessarily led to the elevation of the other senses in instances when sight was deemed unreliable. Certain modern developments – such as the categorization of people according to "race" – were as preoccupied with authenticity as were premodern worries about the essence of a rose's scent and, in both instances, vision was not necessarily preeminent.[18]

Before reconsidering the function of vision during the post-Enlightenment period, it is worthwhile pausing to evaluate the importance of sight during antiquity and the Middle Ages generally not least because doing so suggests that seeing was, in these predominantly Western, non-print cultures, actually quite important.

It is certainly true that many so-called "premodern" societies discounted seeing in some important ways. Early Greek culture, for example, sometimes demonstrated a suspicion of the eye. Wisdom was often sightless and wise men – Homer, Oedipus – were supposedly sightless from birth or blinded later. Similarly, in Norse mythology, Odin traded his sight for wisdom, thus suggesting that not all insight was visual. And, in terms of architecture, although the Greeks certainly paid lots of attention to the optic, they also emphasized the tactile, stressing the texture of materials and the weight of buildings.[19]

While it is certainly the case that the ancient Greeks distinguished quite sharply between the senses and the mind (the former was believed more typical of animals, the latter the provenance of man and reason), it is also true that many Greek thinkers, Plato among them, championed sight as the primary sense. For Plato, vision was the foundation of philosophy, the sense able to convey beauty and, as such, it functioned as the sensory conduit leading to Truth and God.[20] Like Plato, Aristotle also touted the preeminence of sight, linking it to knowledge, but he went a step further and ranked the senses: "Now sight is superior to touch in purity, and hearing and smell to taste." Moreover, Aristotle explained his thinking. Touch, he argued, was the basest, primary sense, belonging to all animals, and, like taste, involved direct physical contact. Touch and taste were also, in his estimation, closely indexed to animal pleasures; conversely, with regard to the senses of sight, hearing, and smell – what he called the "human" senses and ranked in that order – "no one is called profligate if he is in excess." This hierarchy of the senses proved remarkably enduring among intellectuals for centuries and, in this respect, the invention of print and the developments of the Enlightenment appear largely incidental to the rise and empowerment of the eye during and after the Renaissance. The privileging of sight had been conceptualized and elaborated much earlier.[21]

Early Christian thinking about the senses was also highly visualist. While early Christians disagreed on the worth of the senses generally – were they God's munificent gifts or avenues to sin? – sight was often considered preeminent. While all the senses could be avenues for temptation – for John Chrysostom (c. 347–407), the Archbishop of Constantinople, tongues, skin, ears, noses, and eyes were all potentially sinful – the eye was often singled out as more beautiful, powerful, truthful, and godly than the other senses. In the thirteenth century, Saint Thomas Aquinas reaffirmed the Platonic and Aristotelian penchant for sight by giving it pronounced ascetic, religious authority. For Aquinas, "the highest and perfect felicity of intellectual nature consists in the vision of God," not in scent, touch, taste, or sound. As Anthony Synnott has written, "Aquinas gave theological sanction to a long-established philosophical and cultural tradition of the hegemony of sight." Interestingly enough, it was later theologians (including those writing during and after the print revolution), Saint Ignatius Loyola (1491–1536) most obviously, who came increasingly to believe that faith was the basis of truth and eyes could be fooled.[22]

Although the little historical work that has been done on the sensory history of non-Western societies, especially with regard to vision, is from a distinctly philosophical or anthropological perspective and for specific periods only, what research there is suggests a need to qualify claims for the primacy of vision and print and its association with modernity and to appreciate how sight interacted with the other senses to generate intellectual meaning. According to Jane Geaney's analysis of a number of written texts on the epistemology of the senses produced during China's Warring States period (480–221 BCE), for example – a time of social and economic progress in which a politically influential cultural elite emerged from a series of civil wars among competing territories following the collapse of the Zhou Dynasty (c. 1050–256 BCE) – Western sensory hierarchies would have been largely unrecognizable in China. "In contrast to the role of vision in Platonic and Cartesian models of knowing," writes Geaney, neither vision nor hearing was privileged. Certainly, these two senses occupied more prominent places than the others and, in this respect, Chinese sensory epistemology maintained a hierarchy similar to that operational in Western Europe at the same time. But sight and sound in China were wholly parallel and truth and knowledge were deemed contingent on the interaction of both. Reliance on sight alone would not yield true understanding. Moreover, although the Warring States texts often refer to five senses, their number was plastic and often understood in terms less of discrete senses and more in terms of intersensorality and how the senses functioned as a whole.[23]

The social system that emerged in the Warring States period complicated the senses by injecting feudal relations into sensory categories. Thus, while sight and hearing were considered the most reliable senses (or, rather, singular sense, since the two were so tightly braided) generally, China's elites believed that peasants could not be trusted to see and hear properly, their disadvantaged social and economic position undermining the reliability of their eyes and ears. The nobility, by contrast, claimed possession of refined vision and hearing and, as such, were not only the seats of social and political authority but deservedly so, since only elite judgment, mediated by the eyes and ears, could be trusted. Moreover, privilege meant access to technologies that empowered eyes and ears. The "advantage of things like compasses, pitch tubes" and multiple eyes and ears, notes Geaney, "is that they expand the scope of an individual's knowledge," and gave elites who possessed such technologies greater claim over social and territorial authority.[24]

Sight was also critical to Inca religion, at least according to sixteenth-century Spanish sources. Light was an important part of Inca cosmology and creation and it gave definite structure to the secular world, too. The sun was their principle deity and many of the "Inca *huacas* were situated along sight lines radiating out from the central Inca temple." These same lines also helped elaborate social structures by associating different Inca kin with particular lines. In other words, linearity, sight, vision were important to the Inca – a society where modern print was nonexistent and where none of the developments typically associated with hypervisuality had occurred.[25]

So, too, among other South American cultures. Even though the Maya and other Mesoamerican peoples placed heavy emphasis on the importance of smell and hearing, sight was the predominant sense, so much so that even though the three senses were linked in synesthetic fashion it took the stimulus of sight to trigger sound and smell. The principle reason for this emphasis on sight was, perhaps, the centrality of writing – but not print – to Mesoamerican synesthesia. Most script (in the form of speech scrolls) was intended to be read aloud and thus sight and sound were close cousins. Smell figured prominently in courtly life especially. Elites surrounded themselves with flowery fragrances, used them as gifts to subordinates, and thereby associated scent with status. Smells held other significances too, beyond the secular. Flowers and fragrant smells were used not simply to demarcate status or cover stench but floral devices were used to ensure the continued vitality of deceased dignitaries. But even in this society which "regarded sound, odour, and sight in highly concrete ways," with each sense investing "vitality and meaning in the spaces it traversed and occupied," a sensory hierarchy operated with sight at the top or, as with the Chinese example, in tandem with other senses. According to early colonial accounts, religious authority was sometimes represented in depictions of an eyeball which was believed to be not only a receiver of images but generative too, insofar as it established "communion between internal will and external result."[26]

Wither Enlightenment?

Just as pre-Enlightenment Western and non-Western societies could stress the importance and preeminence of the eye without having experienced a McLuhanesque print revolution, so too did the Enlightenment itself have a much more complicated relationship to vision and the other senses than the great divide theory suggests.

In fact, as some recent intellectual historians have shown, nestled in the very guts of the Enlightenment and the Age of Reason, with all its appeals to the beauty, power, and authority of the eye, was a quieter but nonetheless very real preoccupation with non-visual senses which became critically important to the development of modernity in the eighteenth, nineteenth, and twentieth centuries. As Jessica Riskin argues in her recent study, *Science in the Age of Sensibility*, sensoriality was not divorced from the Age of Reason; rather, it was inextricable to it. The basis of knowledge among eighteenth-century French scientists was "sensation and emotion," a sort of "sentimental empiricism" that lent a distinctly emotional and sensory aspect to reason, truth, and knowledge. "Sensory experiences" granted access to knowing and the senses were considered portals to physical and moral science and truth. Riskin shows that debates about the relative power of sight over the other senses (notably Molyneux's Problem which pitted seeing against touch) were central to Enlightenment ideas surrounding scientific truth and intellectual credibility. Sight often won out, to be sure (Denis Diderot considered the sightless "inhumane"), but the putatively lower, premodern sense of touch, for example, was not without its champions, some of whom maintained that it was the sense of the intellect and more likely to reveal truth and depth than the more superficial sense of sight. For instance, in 1800, the physiologist, Philippe Pinel, maintained that "The sense of touch is the sense of the intellect" and it was deemed more reliable than sight in many instances, notably in certain medical treatments. Moreover, Riskin shows that inextricable to the rise of vision were doubts about its reliability, doubts articulated and elaborated by the best Renaissance and Enlightenment minds. In *Meditations* (1641), René Descartes made the case that all of the senses, vision included, were fallible. In other words, even the scientist who did the most to champion the nobility of sight, who applauded the telescope and inventions that empowered the eye as most revealing of truth, preferred to reject the authenticating ability of the eyes – or all the senses – when thinking philosophically. More than that, though, Descartes, who certainly cherished vision, placed a very heavy emphasis on the sense of touch which he believed in some ways "more certain and less vulnerable to error than vision." Similarly, as Roy Porter's magisterial *Flesh in the Age of Reason* shows, eighteenth-century thinking about the essential nature of body and soul was not framed solely in antiseptic, visual terms. Bodies especially were subject to disciplinary protocols elaborated not simply around the way they looked but also how they smelled, felt, and sensed. Ideas about science, society, and truth itself were indexed precisely to the senses and circulated at the center of Enlightenment thinking about the nature of the world.[27]

If we take seriously the argument that the Enlightenment was more sensate and less overpoweringly visual than the great divide theory suggests, we open up theoretical crawlspace to understand how the non-visual senses remained important even as vision became more muscular. Embedded in the Enlightenment were ideas about the enduring value of the other senses, some of which were inherited from antiquity, gestated and reworked during the Enlightenment, and then imported to help from the contours of modernity itself.

Re-Visionist Perspectives II

The great divide theory's tendency to index sight with modernity, to discount the importance of the other senses following the supposedly ocularcentric developments of the print revolution, the Renaissance, and the Enlightenment might not be as tidy as it first suggests. And a number of scholars, especially those interested in the social and cultural history of the senses, have begun to elaborate on this messiness.

Constance Classen, for example, has pointed out how access to and claims upon the higher sense of sight (and, to some extent, hearing) during the Renaissance was very much a gendered issue and should cause us to pause before accepting too enthusiastically claims concerning ways that developments during the Renaissance uniformly elevated the eye. More associated with the lower, proximate senses, women in the West were actively denied access to the ocular. Women's expected roles in the home, nursery, and kitchen were reinforced through their association with the senses of smell, touch, and taste; the sight-oriented activities of men – reading, writing, traveling – were deemed unladylike and women who engaged in such activities (such as the seventeenth-century English writer, Mary Cavendish) were regarded as, at best, quirky, and, at worst, transgressive of gendered norms. In other words, huge swathes of the population were deliberately segregated from the ocular and this exclusion in itself should give us pause before agreeing too heartily that vision experienced such broad authority as the great divide theory suggests. Attending to the sensory components of gender suggests that the great divide theory, rather than having a broad applicability, seems to describe best the shift in sensory ratios among highly literate, elite men and hardly serves as proxy for the experience of large numbers of other people.[28]

The history of medicine also raises questions about the integrity of the great divide theory. It is certainly the case that vision was accorded a prominent role in medicine during and after the eighteenth century. Increasingly, the patient's body was "read," symptoms were recorded in writing, there was an increasing distancing from the body, a tendency not to touch directly, a growing use of anatomical illustration, and a conviction that medical knowledge was mediated primarily through the eye. That much said, this visualism was complicated and the other senses were intimately involved in medical practice. For example, even while the stethoscope helped distance physicians from women and the laboring classes in the nineteenth century – thereby reinforcing sight and diminishing the role of touch – this visual distancing was obviously indebted to the sense of hearing. There were also important continuities between humoral, putatively premodern medicine and "modern" clinical medicine. Consultation remained important to modern doctors; touch was still relevant to both treatment and diagnosis, as was smell, and the medical gaze itself, putatively rational and empirical, often remained hostage to metaphysics and theology.[29]

Some students of the history of Renaissance language and literature have, like some social, cultural, and intellectual historians, also cast serious doubt on the great divide theory and the importance of the print revolution in promoting a supposedly hegemonic way of seeing the world. D. R. Woolf, for example, attends carefully to the relationship between print, orality, and metaphor, arguing: "The frequency of metaphors of sound rather than sight in Renaissance texts suggest that the writers who employed it thought of their works not as silent artifacts to be studied exclusively with the eye, but as instruments for the conveyance of their authorial voice to a public which in turn was conceived of as an audience." As Woolf shows, "the early modern mind was fully capable of balancing aural and visual perception, despite the increased assault on the eyes provided by print" and that "in so doing it merely maintained and developed a 'perceptual equilibrium' present in the later medieval mind rather than shifting from one mode of perception to another." While Woolf does not deny the importance of print in giving rise to visuality, his point that vision, print, and aurality were not mutually exclusive helps explain why people, even after the Enlightenment, continued to listen to the past.[30]

Moreover, during the nineteenth century, vision's power was compromised even as the eye, paradoxically, assumed greater scientific authority. The increasing availability of cheap print and published sources, of spectacles, stereoscopes, daguerreotypes, and photographs; the ability to see at distances never before imagined, the ability to travel to places heretofore largely invisible, the ability to see familiar sights from new perspectives (courtesy of the railroad and balloons), all served to imbue sight with veracity. But even in the midst of assuredness that seeing was believing, other technologies, especially those that rendered the formerly invisible visible (most obviously the increasingly available telescope and microscope), "served to challenge, at the level of popular perception, the quality of observations made by the unaided human eye." Moreover, the Romantic belief in the power of imagination and memory remained a powerful legacy among Victorians, offering another source indicating that the physical act of seeing was subject to a variety of distortions.[31]

As Kate Flint has shown, "The Victorians were fascinated with the act of seeing, with the question of reliability – or otherwise – of the human eye, and with the problems of interpreting what they saw." Nineteenth-century English elites came to question the dominance of sight even as they wanted to believe that seeing was the sense best suited to surveillance, codification, and classification. Critically, Flint shows that even as the belief that the appearance of the body and inner worth could be read by looking at bodies – that types of character were physiologically identifiable – gained popularity, we would be unwise "to assume absolute acceptance by mid-Victorians of these" tenets. The notion that people could dissimilate, mask, and alter the way they looked led many to pause before assigning judgments about character just by looking and, as a result, "identity came to be recognized as something which was not innate, but performative," requiring additional details that were not necessarily visual to authenticate what the eye thought it was seeing.[32]

What was increasingly inscrutable to the eye inspired fear among Victorians. For Londoners, sources of consternation, especially for elites, included class unrest (invisible until too late) and underground sewage (raw material beneath them, always circulating and threatening to escape). The two were not unrelated (both underground, both potentially eruptive) and both held a sensory potency – especially smell – that elites found worrying in its association with disease.

Moreover, smell bombarded from all directions at once while vision gave them perspective and placed things in order. To counteract this fear, English elites attempted to stabilize the invisible and unpredictable by classifying, detailing, describing, and writing a history of certainty on what they found disconcerting, most obviously by giving dangerous things such as workers and sewage systems a communal and visible history in the forms of diagrams and paintings and thereby generating a known past that helped alleviate worries about uncertain futures.[33]

But modern technologies sometimes had a way of exposing the limitations of seeing even as they made heavy use of the eyes. Night was especially problematic for nineteenth-century urban elites because it hid movement and shrouded elements that threatened stability, such as disaffected urban working classes. Modernizers tried to manage nocturnal urban space by introducing gaslight. Gaslight was supposed to make the hours of night as orderly as daytime by making night visible. That it did but, rather than imposing order on nocturnal activities, gaslight often revealed in stark profile the very precariousness of class relations in Victorian London and showed, with brilliant illumination, the effects of rampant industrialism and urban blight. What workers got up to at night – prostitution, ill-disciplined behavior in general, and the general effects of the industrial, modern age – exposed the limits of Victorian modernity, a failing that hit elites squarely in the eye.[34]

Beyond European Eyes

Elsewhere, beyond Europe, doubts about seeing gave rise to a search for additional sensory details in the nineteenth and twentieth centuries. While sight was unsurpassed in being able "to study the vastness and minutiae of the natural world," the other senses played roles in either authenticating or problematizing what was seen.[35]

Take, for example, the history of segregation in the United States, arguably a distinctly modern effort to arrange and categorize people according to the fiction of race and racial identity. But, as the architects of segregation discovered, their very efforts to invent race, to arrange "black" and "white" bodies in public space, exposed the limitations not only of the idea of "race" but of the assumed detectors of racial categories, the eyes.

Revealing examples abound. On March 6, 1907, white residents of the small southern town of Albany, GA, told a man named Peter Zeigler to leave. Zeigler "had been here for a month and palmed himself off as a white man." Citizens had been fooled, even close up: "He has been boarding with one of the best white families in the city and has been associating with some of Albany's best people." Zeigler's luck ran out, it seemed, when "A visiting lady recognized him as being a Negro who formerly lived in her city, and her assertion was investigated and found to be correct." But Zeigler returned to Albany "accompanied by a party composed of relatives and influential friends from his native state of South Carolina" who verified that he was, indeed, white. Peter Zeigler went from being white to black to white because his "race" could not be reliably fixed by the eye of the segregationist.[36]

Instances of "black" people passing into "white" society, of whites mistakenly taking black people as white (or, indeed, taking whites for blacks) were not uncommon in U.S. history. It is tempting to try to understand such instances as illustrating the fundamentally illogical system of segregation, one premised on the putative absolute difference between "black" and "white." But there is more to this matter than, literally, meets the eye. To end analysis with the observation that the Peter Zeigler episode and others like it reveals the operational and intellectual instability of "race" in a period that touted the necessity and existence of racial permanence begs too many pivotal questions. How did such a system recover from such episodes? How did it function for over half a century if it was so fragile, illogical, and built on a distinction that was itself a fiction?

In short, segregationists readily admitted that race could not always be seen, that identity was not always detectable by eye alone. Because segregationists operated in a context that increasingly cast into doubt the reliability of vision as the preeminently authenticating sense, race could not be just visual. New ideas and technologies – photographs, microscopes, germ theory – at once empowered the eye and exposed the limitations of unaided vision. Things small, far, and near could not always be detected or reliably interpreted by the naked eye. Formal segregation was born precisely in a moment that destabilized the idea that seeing was believing.

Witness the very foundation of American, state-sanctioned segregation, *Plessy* v. *Ferguson* (1896). In this case, the U.S. Supreme Court upheld the constitutionality of Louisiana's 1890 statute providing "separate but equal" accommodations for black and white passengers on its railroads. In an event designed to test the 1890 law, Homer Plessy, a visually "white" "black" man (he was seven-eighths "white"), refused to sit in a colored car and was brought before John H. Ferguson, the Judge of the Criminal Court of New Orleans. Plessy's attorney, Albion W. Tourgée argued that because Plessy was visually "white," his race could not be reliably ascertained by the train conductor, the person responsible for sorting out race on a daily basis. The argument that Plessy's race could not be seen held little water with Louisiana's Assistant District Attorney: "I might not be able to see that he is black, but I can certainly smell his racial identity," went the argument. The *Plessy* case profiled an important if often overlooked fact: modern segregation was based on a case involving a black man who was not visibly black, who had to tell whites his race, who told white eyes that vision alone was unreliable when trying to fix and anchor racial identity, and who forced segregationists to maintain that putatively premodern noses were more reliable than eyes when it came to truth claims about racial identity.[37]

Likewise, the widely accepted argument that just one-drop of "African" blood was sufficient to constitute "blackness" – formally embraced by some southern states in the 1920s – reveals the uncertainty of seeing racial identity. After all, the one-drop rule relied on genealogy to ascertain race, not on sight. The one-drop rule itself, then, reveals the lessening relevance of the eye in detecting "race" and to the system of segregation in the late nineteenth and early twentieth centuries.[38]

In short, the system of segregation relied on what white southerners – white Americans generally – believed were the detective powers of non-visual senses – taste, touch, smell, hearing – to locate the thing they constructed as "race." Some of the time, they thought they could see racial identity and when they could not, they happily appealed to their other senses to help verification. Of course, the sensory fixing of race – itself a fiction – was far from perfect simply because race itself was (and remains) a construction. Black people did not have an innately distinctive odor, did not have a genetically coded "sound," did not have a racially determined texture to their skin. The likes of Peter Ziegler showed as much. But segregationists lived with the chance of missing the Peter Zeiglers of their world (if, in fact, he was "black") and convinced themselves that race was, on the whole, detectable in deep, emotional ways to all of the senses.[39]

Clearly, then, if sight did triumph in the nineteenth and twentieth centuries, it did so very unevenly and often dragged "premodern" sensory beliefs and superstitions with it well into the twentieth century. For example, artificial lighting in Russian cities, first introduced in the 1850s, took a long time to be accepted by many Russians as something good, reliable, and authentic. Early gas and, later, electric lighting was associated with the devil, an image popularized in peasant folklore and by Russia's literati. If Jerusalem could rely on the sun and

God's light alone, so too could St. Petersburg, they reasoned. Many Russians considered "Electric suns," as street lights were known in the 1850s, ungodly and unnatural, contrary to the natural and divinely ordained light of the sun. Rather than offering reliable perspective and illumination, they understood street lights as "unnatural, dead and inanimate." Human faces, some Russians claimed in 1878, "do not have their natural healthy appearance" in such light. Artificial light was just that: false and hardly revealing of truth. Street lights were deceptive, infernal, and underhand and under their glare places like St. Petersburg seemed sinister and dangerous – hardly enlightened places. Artificial light eventually became accepted, of course, but it took time. According to Andrei Toporkov, it was not until the mid-twentieth century that the Russian city dweller "became a pragmatist who demanded only one thing of the street lamp: that it light pavement and road for people, buses and cars at night."[40]

In fact, the specific histories of individual cities suggests the heuristic limitations of talking about a broadly understood and homogenous "reception" of seeing and light under modernity. As Samuel Martland's work shows, although nineteenth-century Valparaiso and Santiago in Chile and La Plata in Argentina all embraced street lighting as an "eminently flexible strategy of modernization," the precise meaning of illuminated vision, light, and night in each city varied considerably. While all three cities introduced bright, ornate, and inexpensive street lights as the "most visible antidote to the sense of inferiority that many elite Latin Americans felt towards European and North American cities," each city understood street lights and their visual meaning differently. The port city of Valparaiso, for example, was a town of narrow streets with a topography that appeared to give cover to nocturnal criminal behavior, a perception strengthened by the obvious presence of foreign sailors and migrants. Here, pragmatic concerns guided the installation of street lights in the nineteenth century. The police lobbied for them, property owners wanted them, and basic economic demands that the streets function as safe arteries of travel dictated lighting the night. In Argentina's planned city of La Plata, by contrast, street lights functioned purely as an esthetic and ideological statement: they were there to claim the city and, by extension, the country, as modern. Santiago was a blend of both: there, lights claimed modernity but also functioned as a tool of social control, allowing officials to police behavior and combat crime. In other words, the historical experience of seeing, the wide variety of ways in which light was understood, experienced, and used suggests the limitations of a great divide theory that places undue weight on the invention and dissemination of print culture as the principal explanation for a development – the triumph of vision – which has a messier, more convoluted, contingent, and complicated history than any broad-brush theory allows.⁴¹

2

Hearing

Look, Hear: Listening

In their attentiveness to the heard worlds of the past, many historians, myself included, have sometimes echoed the traditional hierarchy of the senses: quantitatively, historical work on hearing is second only to work on sight. Hearing, the sense in much of Western history most commonly assumed to bridge the "highest" sense of sight and the "lower" senses of smell, taste, and touch, has received quite sustained examination from intellectual and social-cultural historians (at least for the West). Such attention to aurality, though, has been beneficial not least because work on hearing, listening, and sound has complicated the easy association between sight, sound, print, and modern and premodern eras. As a number of recent studies have shown, important aspects of modernity were deeply indebted to aurality during and after the Enlightenment in the West and in non-Western societies too.[1]

That much said, we are, for several reasons, still some way from a thorough understanding of the historical importance of sound and aurality. First, the great divide theory's reliance on orality, thanks to the heavy emphasis on the printed and heard word and the interpretive weight placed on that moment of historical transition between the two, privileges orality and linguistic sounds over aural, paralinguistic, and non-vocable sounds – the sounds of the mundane and everyday originating outside of the mouth. Second, a good deal of aural history is driven by a music-centered framework. For example, while Jacques Attali's framework for understanding the history of sound is not as influential as that of Ong and McLuhan's, it has nevertheless shaped the ways in which some historians think about sound. In short, Attali's work serves to wed sound to music in ways that, while interesting and profitable at some level, nevertheless entertain an unnecessarily limited view of sound as music. In his book, *Noise: The Political Economy of Music*, Attali outlined how changes in music foreshowed historical changes in economy and polity. Attali sequenced music and stages – sacrifice, representation, repetition, and composing – to suggest how, for example, music functioned as sacrifice typically in ancient societies. Such societies, he maintains, lived in a state of fear with music increasingly serving as a simulacrum or substitute for violence. Attali also claimed that the vocabulary for discussing music became increasingly credentialized and owned by aficionados, not the masses.[2] Yet Attali too promotes a similar privileging because he tends to treat music as the *sine qua non* of sound. As Douglas Kahn has pointed out, the consistent privileging of music as the art of sound in modern Western culture has made efforts to listen outside of that rubric difficult and frustrating. Music continually intervenes, uninvited, as the legitimate site and standard of (aurally mediated) art and crowds out all sorts of other sounds.[3] This chapter takes Kahn's point seriously and, as such, attends much less to music (although it is not unmindful of the topic) and much more to work on the history of sound, construed broadly, and taken to include noise and silence too.

Echoes from the "Premodern" West, and Beyond

There is no doubt that McLuhan and Ong were quite right to stress that the absence of the printed word in particular societies, especially those in the pre-Enlightenment West, had the effect of making sound and the heard world extremely important not only for communication but also for arranging, affirming, and mediating various forms of social organization and hierarchy.

The spoken and heard word figured prominently in legal proceedings and arrangements in many premodern Western societies. In Rome (5 BCE) parties bound themselves with the spoken word while land transfers in tenth-century England were uttered, their "saying mattered more than the writing." Non-vocable sounds were also integral to legal culture. According to Bernard Hibbitts, "Early medieval contracts were often made by the buyer slapping the palm of the seller, an action that seems to have been calculated for aural as much as physical effect."[4]

In societies where writing played little or no substantive role, cultures of sound and hearing predominated. According to Hibbitts, "Performative wisemen are primarily talkers, not writers. Socrates, one of the last Greek sages to live in a performative environment, never wrote down any of his thoughts." As late as the fourth century BCE,

Plato equated hearing with knowledge and understanding. Sound was also essential for establishing political, social, and religious space. The Greek polis was sometimes delimited by the range of the crier's voice, as were Medieval European villages (larger towns were subdivided into wards according to hearing distances), a practice that proved enduring – Christian parishes, in Europe and colonial America, were often defined by the distance at which church bells could be heard.[5]

Sound was important even in word-oriented circumstances and areas where writing (though not, obviously, print) mattered. Exaggerated reports concerning early Christian asceticism notwithstanding, sensory delights were important to early Christian worship. For example, oral and aural senses were gratified by the chanting of the liturgy. Sound, voice, and hearing were important to faith and the spiritual significance of sound was frequently reflected in the acoustic architecture of early Christian churches in the East and West. And according to the notion of the music of the spheres – the sound of heaven occasionally interrupted by the noise of the devil – planetary movement itself was regulated by sound and music. Hearing also played an important role in medicine, especially in the Galenic diagnosis of disease in ancient Greece. Physicians listened not only to the patient's words describing their condition – typical of Galenic consultation – but also listened to the body itself.[6]

The importance of sound and hearing to the ancient and medieval world becomes apparent when we consider how early written records attempted to capture the importance of spoken words. Wills, for example, were often spoken at the point of death. Here, we can hear an eleventh-century English will recorded in the *Domesday* Book: "Hark, my friends. I will that my wife shall hold this land which I bought from the Church as long as she lives." Making a will "with his mouth" was quite typical in England down to the thirteenth century. Moreover, all sorts of orally communicated legal pronouncement remained common throughout Medieval Europe. Town criers, just as they had under the Roman Republic, announced statutes and decrees. Indeed, in Medieval Iceland, the word for "legal claim" and "speech" were the same. Such oral and aural communication was most often an urban matter. Town criers – and the laws they announced – were most audible to the greatest number of people in urban areas, less so in the countryside.[7]

Unsurprisingly, questions of aurality – especially how sound was produced and heard and the actual and metaphorical meanings attributed to hearing – were considered at great length by a variety of thinkers during the Middle Ages. Much of their thinking was based on the work of ancient philosophers, Aristotle principally. Charles Burnett's important work has shown how philosophers ranging from Aristotle to Albertus Magnus identified sound, understood how it was propagated, and debated how sound was perceived. Few hard answers were forthcoming, suggests Burnett. "The dominant impression one gets from reading medieval philosopher's accounts of sound," he remarks, "is their fascination with the illusiveness of the entity," mainly because there was a widespread recognition that actual hearing was often deceptive and not as reliable as sight in identifying truth. Doubts about the reliability of hearing notwithstanding, serious thinkers devoted enough time and effort trying to fathom the nature of sound and hearing to accord the sense great importance, often second only to sight in the medieval sensory hierarchy.[8]

Ancient and medieval theories of hearing proved remarkably enduring even after the print revolution, as Penelope Gouk has shown in her work on seventeenth-century England. Gouk highlights the influence of ancient philosophers on a number of English thinkers in their discussions concerning natural philosophy and sound and sound's relationship to the mind, soul, body, and the natural world. Aristotelian ideas about sound remained popular in sixteenth- and seventeenth-century thought, especially the notion that sound was a product of two bodies striking against one another. His comparison of sound to water waves also retained currency. Anatomical investigations based on a reading of Aristotle also became important. Helkiah Crooke's *Microcosmographia*, published in 1615, offered a very early anatomical account of hearing which both echoed Aristotle and invested hearing with considerable intellectual authority. Crooke followed Aristotle in two respects. First, he attempted to explain the effects of music on the listener by claiming that music excited and stirred up the spirits in and about the heart, making the listener tremble. Second, again agreeing with Aristotle, he postulated that while seeing was the most functional and necessary of the senses for securing the needs and wants in life, things that were heard impressed the mind and intellect more deeply than objects that were seen.[9]

Beyond the association between intellect and hearing, sound was plainly critical to daily life in early modern Europe. Throughout towns, sounds served to coordinate civic, political, economic, and social life. Sounds functioned as a semiotic system, helping people locate themselves in space as well as time, with familiar sounds and their timing helping to establish the idea of community. Variations in urban soundscapes abounded, naturally. For example, bells tolled for death everywhere but in some towns, smaller bells were used for children and women and louder ones for men, especially those of rank. Town criers, market voices, shouts, as well as non-vocal sounds – the rattling of carriages, the clopping of horses, the sounds of particular bells that, from Moscow to Dublin, gave each city a distinctive aural signature, the tap of hammers and hiss of forges – all served not only to give early modern European towns a broadly understood urban soundscape but, simultaneously, keynotes peculiarly their own.[10]

How sounds served to locate and identify place, class and, increasingly, national identity in the early modern period – and how, as we'll see, sounds performed very similar functions in the modern era – suggests how hearing operated in conjunction with seeing. For example, economic development could be heard as well as seen in sixteenth-century London. Not only could the sound of business, trade, and economic productivity be loud – and increasingly so to contemporaries generally – but formerly discrete soundscapes where the sounds of one trade were limited to a particular geographic area collapsed, spilling their sounds into adjacent streets and regions. Economic development was marked, then, by a mixing of sounds – the sounds of the cooper blending with those of the smith – and so the sound of industriousness was heard not simply in the cadence and register of one trade but in the acoustic braiding of many. If economic development in early modern London was increasingly loud, noisy, even cacophonous, these very soundmarks also came to identify Londoners specifically, the English generally, as having a distinctive sound, at least to foreign ears. Visitors from continental Europe described sixteenth- and seventeenth-century Londoners as lovers of noise – their fondness for booming cannon, ringing bells, and beating drums earning particular comment – and understood part of the English character in acoustemological terms. That is, unless, these same travelers visited royalty. Here, class and status intervened: the Crown, nobles generally, counterpoised themselves against the masses by embracing quietude, not loudness. The interior furnishings of court – carpets, curtains, and the like – muted noises, the monarch's voice was the supreme sound, and everyone modulated their own sounds accordingly. In this way, the ability to afford and insist on quietude became increasingly associated with class and notions of refinement and taste.[11]

Acoustic markers of place, identity, and class migrated with Europeans as they colonized North America. As Richard Rath has shown in his remarkable study of soundways in early America, sound and ways of hearing were used to regulate, create, and arrange social hierarchies and define and extend social and cultural authority. He shows, for example, how the spatial and acoustic properties of churches and meeting houses reflected and reaffirmed political and social ordering. Rath's discussion of churches and chapels in the sixteenth- and seventeenth-century Chesapeake, Virginia, especially, reveals with wonderful clarity the importance of hearing to religious worship and the establishment of social hierarchy. Anglicans in the Chesapeake, not unlike their English forebears, designed chapels that raised the minister up high so that his words could be heard. Sounding boards were also used to concentrate his voice and amplify it, giving his voice volume and authority. But not every one in the congregation heard equally. Those in the front – usually the wealthiest and of high social standing in this increasingly slave-based, plantation society – had best access to the minister's voice; those at the back in galleries, frequently the poor and, later in the period, the enslaved, could not hear his voice as well and, by implication, found their pastoral needs, their faith, and their religious beliefs discounted. Sound and hearing indexed status as well as faith in early America, even as the print revolution was beginning to make its presence felt.[12]

The pre-Enlightenment West's stress on the importance of hearing was shared by many non-Western societies. Non-literate or partially literate societies everywhere seem to have placed great importance on aurality. We know that sound played a critical role in the Hindu tradition during the Vedic period (1500–700 BCE), for example, with vibration holding meaning independently of vision. And, as in Europe, even when texts began to capture meaning, sound retained enormous currency. Similarly, Inca cosmologies recorded after the Spanish Conquest in the sixteenth century show that orality and hearing occupied an important place in religious practice and theology. Inca priests were believed to have the power to make things talk, and hearing, too, was thoroughly implicated in Incan secular and religious life. Echoes remain. "Many Andeans today," writes Constance Classen, "look nostalgically back on the pre-Conquest period as a golden aural/oral age when the world was animated by sound." As Classen maintains, their past was more aurally and orally centered.[13]

In more secular terms, sound was (and, according anthropological work, still is) used in a variety of non-Western societies to define political and social territory and communicate all manner of information. This was especially the case with "drum languages," used in many places, but in West Africa especially. Historically, communication in West Africa was "overwhelmingly sonic" and drums, whistles, horns, and yodeling were used to convey information between communities that were beyond eye-shot. The nature of this communication was complicated and subtle, relying heavily on fluctuations in pitch, tone, and rhythm and sometimes as involved as some written forms of communication. Such communicative technologies were also extremely adaptable and able to resist the worst excesses of seventeenth and eighteenth century imperialism and capitalism, retaining, as they did, enormous importance among the New World's enslaved population who used drums and other aural forms of communication not only to preserve their cultural values but also to resist bondage and, at times, coordinate revolts.[14]

Moreover, lots of aurally inclined societies located intellect in the heard as well as the seen world. According to George Devereux's research, the tendency to "equate speech with intelligence" was typical in classical Malay: "In ancient Malay speech or words in general seem to have been deemed the chief means of activity." The Sedant Moi of Indochina also considered the ear the seat of intellect and reason and a similar auralcentrism prevailed in Buddhist iconography – sages were often depicted as having large ears. Devereux's research specifically, and work on ancient non-Western societies generally (little though there is, regrettably), are fascinating because they help blur the distinction between Western European and Asiatic sensory cultures and the histories that produced them. Societies (European and Malay) equating speech with intelligence, Devereux maintains, might be best understood as "self-oriented, mastery seeking," with a developed sense of self that is imposed onto reality. Hearing societies, conversely, embraced a more passive, self-less understanding of the individual and the world where the primacy of the sense of hearing merges the self with the world. Thus, societies that profile hearing rather than seeing will likely have a different history, especially with regard to the emergence of ideas concerning selfhood.[15]

For largely environmental and historical reasons, some societies placed more emphasis on sound than on sight. As Steven Feld's important ethnographic work on the Kaluli shows, the limited sight-lines and visual scope of the Kaluli environment (the tropical rainforests of Papua New Guinea) historically made them much more dependent on sound to communicate, so much so that sounds and words came to assume powerful spiritual meaning and, in some important ways, constituted Kaluli cultural expression itself. Kaluli acoustemology was (and remains) sufficiently versatile and powerful to function not simply as a way to communicate in the forest but to articulate the connections bridging the visible and invisible, secular and religious worlds. For the

Kaluli, sound was, arguably, the preeminent sense giving meaning to their worlds.[16]

Sounds "Modern"

If hearing and sound remained important in the early modern period in Europe at precisely the point when print culture was beginning to spread and all of its associated visual conceits were beginning to sink into a general consciousness, we might reasonably expect the modern era to have diluted the emphasis on hearing, especially as print culture joined with Renaissance science and Enlightenment rationalism to promote seeing in a more robust way than the developments of the early modern period alone could achieve. But as a lot of work on sound and hearing in the eighteenth, nineteenth, and twentieth centuries makes clear, this was not the case. Hearing and sound remained critical to the elaboration of modernity.

Virtually all the evidence produced by historians of aurality and hearing of the modern era points to a continued importance of hearing and, implicitly at least, heavily discounts the effect print had on diluting aurality in favor of sight. For example, hearing was key to developments in medicine. René-Théophile-Hyacinthe Laënnec's stethoscope was invented in 1816 and "mediated auscultation established itself as a more successful auditory penetrant than percussion." As E. Valentine Daniel explains, auscultation "heralds in the objective physician in a quite dramatic way" because it enabled him to objectify the patient using sound (just as with his gaze). Daniel explains: "No longer is it necessary for the physician to get snarled in and by the patient's experiences and symptoms; instead, he is able to isolate himself from the patient's 'noises' and listens to the sounds produced in the patient, sounds to which the patient has no access and over which he has little control." Moreover, because stethoscopy did not involve direct contact with the patient's body, increasingly professional men did not need to touch either the laboring classes or modest ladies. Stethoscopy and hearing distanced bodies and allowed remote diagnoses.[17]

Just as it had begun to in the early modern period, sound increasingly mediated and helped inform ideas about class, identity, and nationalism, especially, in the nineteenth century. A good deal of writing on aurality in the modern period has been centered on the experience of France which might, as Alain Corbin suggested, stand as broad proxy for the Western experience generally. Specifically, Corbin identified shifts in thresholds of hearing (mainly through his study of bells) that were often class based with people in the countryside clashing with urbanites not only over the meaning of peals and bells but on their timing and use. "Complaining of the discomfort caused by the din of bells was a venerable *urban tradition*," writes Corbin, "and one that fits with the familiar theme of the drawbacks of town life. It formed part of a struggle of the elites, who were intent on imposing their fastidious tastes and reducing noise to some sort of harmonious order, against 'rough music,' charivaris, and rackets, which all served to define the people." In this class conflict resided a dispute over religion and nationalism: "The leaders of the First Republic had sought to desacralize these instruments, to limit their strictly religious uses, to curb their sensory ascendancy, and to monopolize their solemnity. They also attempted to secularize and municipalize the peals, to subordinate them to the nation, and to insert them into a framework of citizenship" and, in effect, "to alter the prevailing pattern" of the culture of the senses and the social hierarchies shaping that culture.[18]

The idea that sound and aurality influenced national and class identity was not peculiar to France. The first half of the nineteenth century in the United States, for example, was characterized by increasing sectional tensions between a free wage labor, largely democratic North and a slave-based South. Sounds anchored and helped define each region and each section trumpeted its soundmarks as at once distinctive and desirable. Northerners applauded the hum of industrialism and, for the most part, the healthy chatter of (limited) democracy while castigating southern slavery as an ominously silent, backward society, where only the cries of whipped slaves punctured the sinister quiet. Southern slaveholders countered by casting their hierarchical society as reassuringly quiet, a place where order was both heard and inspired by careful attention to sounds and their timing. The slaveholders also listened northward and considered the sounds emanating from the North "noises" indicative of imminent social revolution produced by a reckless embrace of liberal capitalism. The integrity of the American nation-state was secured only after the country fought a very bloody civil war (one that had its own soundscapes). Both sections sounded increasingly similar after the Civil War, not least because the keynote of slavery had been silenced by Northern military victory.[19]

Sound was implicated in other nationalist movements, sometimes in impossibly grim ways. German nationalism, for example, was heavily indebted to sounds, and not just those made and theorized by Wilhelm Richard Wagner and Theodor Adorno. Nicholas Vazsonyi has revealed, for example, the critical role played by Enlightenment music in elaborating German culture. In Mozart's *Die Zauberflöte* (*The Magic Flute*, 1791), he finds a connection between "the German enlightenment project" and "the building of a German nation" and locates a "darker" nationalist impulse in German music even at the height of Enlightenment ideals in the late eighteenth century. Later, in the twentieth century, cinematic sound was critical to the formation and elaboration of Nazi identity. Nazi officials understood it as a "viable means to disseminate the timbre of the German language and German musical tradition, and, in doing so, to integrate diverse viewers into the national community." "In the view of Nazi film officials," note Nora M. Alter and Lutz Koepnick, "sound thus not only constituted the modern mass as mass, but also naturalized the community of viewers/listeners into something primordial." In other words, "Sonic material was often essential to the foundation of authoritarian rule and the segregation of cultural identities in modern Germany."[20]

But the eighteenth and nineteenth centuries – the modern era generally – were not all about sound and noise. Silence occupied an important – and telling – place. "Silence too has a history," rightly argues Joy Parr, although one would be hard pressed to find it in some historiographies, most of which detect historical action and agency through the active making of sound, not silence. Yet listening for moments of silence and the redefinition of noise and sound can reveal pivotal shifts in the political realm and social structure.[21]

"All public expression of musical response – even silence – is inevitably social," argues James H. Johnson who shows how, between 1750 and 1850, French theater audiences stopped talking, became quieter, and started listening. Johnson charts the emergence of a "new way of listening ... at the end of the Old Regime, one more attuned to sentiments and emotions in the music and more engaged esthetically than mid-century audiences has described." Audiences now responded to, and listened for, passion in music. The identification of what Johnson calls the "more emotional stratum of musical expression" encouraged spectators "to turn inward to feel the passions the music evoked." To appreciate fully the emotional texture of music meant that one had to focus and remain less distracted socially which, according to Johnson, amounted to a new esthetic appreciation. Such a new mode of listening – active hearing and judging – was at once both intensely subjective but also collective, replete with public and political meaning, not least because the new habit "effectively challenged traditional absolutist patterns of judgment by offering a third source of musical arbitration apart from both the king and the opinion of disconnected groups." But even as such a process trumpeted a more egalitarian sensibility, Johnson shows how the rise of silent spectators served to define bourgeois sensibilities, confirm social identity, police manners, and, in the process, exclude (and define) social "others." Injunctions for silence became markers of class, authority, and taste.[22]

For other eighteenth- and nineteenth-century elites, such injunctions were rooted in an older, more hierarchical view of the world, one in which ruling classes demanded quietude in an effort to reaffirm in daily fashion the contours of power in their society. This more hierarchical use of sound – and silence – is quite apparent in nineteenth century slave societies. Antebellum American slaveholders, for example, cherished a worldview marked by obedience from their inferiors and dependents – slaves, obviously, but women and children too – and used sound and silence to gauge how readily that world was realized on a daily basis. Slaveholders insisted on quietude on their plantations because that preferred soundscape fed, in precise and meaningful ways, their understanding of social order. Slaveholders considered themselves maestros, sculpting the sounds of their world precisely and purposefully. Laboring slaves in cotton fields were supposed to sing, their songs and cadence feeding the planter's conceits about efficiency and productivity. Slaves at rest were, ideally, quiet slaves, calm slaves, composed and obedient. Slaveholders embraced these social ideals enthusiastically and, at least in part, expressed them in aural terms.[23]

The enslaved contested such efforts, however. Sometimes, they countered by offering alternative soundscapes, ones meaningful to, and made by, them. What for white ears was jumbled cacophony, black ears heard as expressive of African American cultural values.[24] The enslaved also used silence and quietude itself to resist. Not all slave religious practices were loud and bondpeople frequently prayed into upturned pots and damp blankets (which either contorted or absorbed their sounds). Slaves also learned to use stealth and silence to escape bondage. Successful runaways often escaped because they understood the value of remaining silent, knowing how to walk silently, and using the very value their masters cherished – quiet – to extricate themselves from slavery.[25]

In less constrained societies, especially under burgeoning nineteenth-century democracies, religious enthusiasm and faith was very much a heard, loud affair. That much said, power and authority was contested aurally and different denominations and faiths used sound to define themselves and denigrate others. As Leigh Eric Schmidt has shown in his marvelous study of evangelical Christianity in America, different classes and social groups contested the meaning of religious sounds.

"Evangelicals were noisy – to their opponents appallingly so," maintains Schmidt. Antirevivalists such as Charles Chauncy used the charge of noise to construct and demarcate otherness, including women and slaves, and, by default, to describe sober, quieter forms of praise as more sincere and refined. Loud voices indicated dull ears, said Chauncy, and only attentive listeners who offered carefully modulated praise had true faith. Anything less was the product of misguided lower orders whose inferiority could be heard in the volume and timbre of their styles of worship.[26]

Yet the very idea that religion and faith could have had such an important aural component to it is difficult to grasp if we place undue emphasis on the notion that the Enlightenment elevated the eye and denigrated the ear. As Schmidt remarks, "It would be wrong ... to turn too quickly to Enlightenment regimens and away from these sound Christians. Extraordinary calls ... continued to flourish in popular Protestant piety, and evangelical ways of hearing hardly lost their resonance; if anything, they radiated ever more widely in modernity's wake." For, as Schmidt shows, while Christian devotionalism generally had always appealed to aurality to mark faith and explain the soul, popular evangelicalism increasingly served "as an inlet into a piety of intimate voices that was, by turns, relished and reviled." To the conservative Old Lights and men such as Chauncy – who well understood the larger relevance of the sense of hearing to faith – evangelicalism was noisy, undercutting the reverence of faith expressed in silence, and disruptive of social hierarchies. Evangelical noise was worrying precisely because the sounds of revivals were invasive, made often by the poor, women, and slaves, and could not be contained. For evangelicals, however, the heard, disembodied voice of God served as a way to make sense of his immutability while at the same time giving rise to demonstrative revival meetings whose volume served to call together potential converts. Thus, argues Schmidt, alongside the controlling restraints of Enlightenment theology traveled a powerful, aural force that in its democratic aspects embodied keynotes of American modernity while also serving to profile the tensions inherent in its evolution.[27]

Modernity generally was as much about trying to control sound as producing it and industrialization and urbanization upped the ante in this regard. As environmental historian, Raymond Smilor, has shown, the period 1893–1932 witnessed shifts in what was deemed productive and unproductive noise and saw a reclaiming of the desirability of relative silence and quietude in some North American cities. Urban elites considered the sounds of machinery and of the working classes in the late nineteenth century inextricable to modernity and a necessary part of capitalist progress. Early twentieth century reformers of the Progressive Era, however, reconstituted the sound of modernity into the noise of modernity, painting not just the clamor of workers but also clanking machinery as atavistic, "inefficient," and premodern. They tried to deal with noisy modernity in all its forms by launching anti-noise campaigns and defining through legislation what constituted social noise. They criticized the working classes as noisy and called for automobiles and various machines to be fitted with quiet ball bearings, gears, and better oil in an effort to dampen the excessive noise of the modern – the very thing northern elites of an earlier generation had applauded.[28]

Progressive Era urban anti-noise campaigns, mostly in northern cities, were important not just for redefining the nature of noise but for reconfiguring how people thought about the sounds of modernity. Whereas an earlier antebellum generation applauded the hum of industry and lambasted the silence of slavery, reformers now, fifty or so years later, identified similar noises as damaging to American progress. Cooperation in combating noise cut across class lines, argues Smilor, not least because "noise was a problem that affected everyone intimately." Bourgeois reformers embraced sound – "activity, work and progress" – while deploring noise, which they believed "signaled waste, disorder and regression," something that disturbed sleep and threatened mental and physical health. Noise was cast as primitive and damaging to the quiet of civilization.[29]

Similar conversations about noise and its meaning and management took place elsewhere, including Germany and, most notably, Victorian London, where the middle classes attempted to remove what they construed as the noise of working class music from the streets and, in the process, preserve English culture from the contaminating noise of foreigners, the lower orders, and the debilitating effects of modern urban life generally. These concerns were especially important to an emerging class of Victorian intellectuals and professionals who coveted quiet for its assumed ability to inspire the *vita comtemplativa*. Noise was, then, not just a public health issue for these professionals. They objected less because their rest and leisure were disturbed by the noise of the lower orders – although that was an important consideration – and more because noise undermined the very nature of their mental labor and national identity.[30]

Legal and social efforts to combat the sounds of modernity foundered on the very subjectivity of defining what was noise and what was sound. Architecture, though, was rather more successful at combating noise because architects apparently enjoyed a more stable definition of sound and necessary and unnecessary noise, especially in working environments. As Emily Thompson has shown in her fine study, *The Soundscape of Modernity*, which charts a culture of listening and how that culture was influenced by architectural acoustics in America, 1900–1933, building modernity itself created din. While municipal and state-sponsored organizations such as New York's Noise Abatement Commission tried to eliminate noise "without much success," Thompson shows how architectural acoustics and scientific technology managed to control noises within buildings and, in the process, altered the relationship between space and sound and Americans' understanding of modernity. By charting the rise of "the business of sound control," exploring the manufacturing of acoustical building materials, and by revealing how architects incorporated these materials into the buildings they designed, Thompson shows how these materials "didn't simply eliminate noises of the modern era, they additionally created a new, modern sound of their own."[31]

These material changes and technological innovations were partnered by "new trends in the culture of listening" which helped constitute modernity in twentieth-century America. The sounds and the esthetics of listening were deemed modern because they involved a rejection of unnecessary sounds and an embrace of a purer, signal-generated, direct sound. The new sounds in office buildings lacked reverberation. Reverberated sound was noise because it was inefficient, interfered with the clear transmission of sound (and speech), and "also impeded the performance of work by amplifying and sustaining the cacophony of sounds that sapped workers' energy and productivity." Absorptive materials were modern because they helped muffle and contain reverberation and increase efficiency. As Thompson explains: "When reverberation was reconceived as noise, it lost its traditional meaning as the acoustic signature of a space, and the age-old connection between sound and space – a connection as old as architecture itself – was severed." With advances in acoustic technology, consumers could buy quiet and come close to banishing certain types of noise from within their homes. All of this was understood as modern because "it was perceived to demonstrate man's technical mastery over his physical environment." Moreover, this was achieved by dint of market, not government, forces, with consumer demand leading the way.[32]

The other main development in the West that serves not only to illustrate the importance of sound and hearing under modernity but, in fact, suggests the increasing instability of the eye at the end of the nineteenth and early decades of the twentieth centuries concerns recorded sound. If actual sounds were ephemeral, what was the impact of the ability to record sound? First, it is important to note that far from being permanent, early wax records were fragile, their principal form of durability residing in the minds of what historian Jonathan Sterne styles as an "emergent culture of preservation." Yet records gave the appearance of permanence, capturing sounds and words that had theretofore seemed fleeting and that could be fixed, however unsatisfactorily, only by script and print. The advent of recorded sound, then, was an important cultural and technological development with significant implications for our understanding of hearing and its relationship to vision at the beginning of the twentieth century.[33]

For example, as Lisa Gitelman's work on the rise of recorded sound in early twentieth-century America has shown, "the new technology of recorded sound helped to challenge the visual habits of musical practice." Gitelman reveals how "the shifting optics of popular music brought pressure to bear on other visual habits, including associations between racial difference and skin color." Record companies – entities sponsoring the commercial recording and capturing of the voice – helped accelerate a racial politics of sound, popularized the idea of the disembodied voice, and separated race from the eye and thereby endorsed the notion that racial identity could be heard, sold, and consumed. The emergence of recorded sound destabilized the relationship between seeing music performed (and reading its texts) and hearing music and, in the process, promoted an essentialist definition of race. Records – and their marketing – invited serious questions. Was that the voice of a black or white singer? Was there a racial signature to a style of music? And what did the attempt to hear "race" in voice say about the listener? Visuality remained important, not least because record producers used sight to either reaffirm or disrupt the relationship between sound and race, but the net effect was to embolden a socially acceptable and nation-wide aural dimension to race at precisely the moment when those championing the separation of the races were searching for non-visual ways to authenticate racial identity. Audiences increasingly "interrogated records as racialized performances," separating the seeing and hearing of racial identity and, in the process, helped establish race as a thoroughly sensory category, one beyond the eye but (supposedly) detectable by the ear. Moreover, recorded sound proved especially alluring to intellectuals, particularly anthropologists who fancied that they could capture for the future what they heard as the sounds of dying cultures – the sounds and music of Native Americans, especially. But in the very process of recording Native American sounds, late nineteenth-century anthropologists, like the earliest commercial recoding companies, served to further demarcate the distinction between white American culture and the culture of the Indian other.[34]

Colonizing Sounds

Aurality, meanings of sound, ways of hearing were part and parcel of the cultural baggage European adventurers, explorers, and colonizers took with them on miscellaneous – and deadly serious – imperial quests beginning in the sixteenth century. Europeans exported well-honed sound technologies (often of medieval origin) and the new commercial and capitalistic cultural values underwriting them to discipline the bodies of natives, principally to exploit their labor but also to tattoo authority on colonized bodies via their ears.

This process can be seen in any number of colonial societies and in each the bell, allied with the clock, was often present. The sound of time, in short, stood in the vanguard of colonialism. In nineteenth-century South Africa, for example, European settlers used clock-regulated bells to introduce Natal natives, mainly Zulus, to ideas concerning wage labor, efficiency, and bodily discipline. In towns especially – public clock time was established in Durban in 1860 – European capitalists, intent on making disciplined laborers out of agricultural Africans who embraced a more flexible and less regimented sense of time, ran schools, civic affairs, and labor by the sound of clock-defined time. The use of public time and bells that had begun in earnest in early modern Europe was imported into the nineteenth century colonial, capitalist mindset and then re-exported around the globe. It took time and effort to instill a sense of time-discipline among Africans in Natal and many resisted the clock and its aural courier, preferring instead to work on their terms at their pace – not unlike workers and servants in eighteenth- and nineteenth-century Europe, North America, and South America who waged similar struggles against the factory bell and what it represented at roughly the same time. But the sound of time and the wage labor economy that it regulated took its toll – as bells often do – and many Natal Africans found themselves firmly ensconced in clock-regulated capitalist social and economic relations by the end of the nineteenth century.[35]

While a similar process seems to have unfolded elsewhere, notably in Australia where colonizers attempted to use clock-regulated bells to discipline not only the nascent Australian working classes but also aboriginal people, the function of sound in the process of colonial encounter in Australia is revealing in other ways. Here, the role of sound in the imperial and colonial project was not simply about imposing authority on various native and aboriginal peoples; it was also about the definition of selves and the formation of new national identities. As Paul Carter explains in his fascinating study, *The Sound In-Between*, we need to "augment the eye with the ear" to understand the Australian past. Carter examines the history of the "word-sound" "Cooee," a sound now understood as quintessentially (white) Australian. But its history has everything to do with claiming ownership of a sound, its appropriation, and its incorporation. European definitions of the word differed markedly from Aboriginal ones. Explains Carter: "the Aboriginal 'Cooee' criss-crossed a space where people felt at home, the European 'Cooee' was cast out into the unknown, a voice crying in the wilderness." In the late 1800s, Europeans adopted Cooee – and abandoned "hallo" – not for any cultural reasons but for purely physical ones: pronouncing Cooee "produced a greater volume of sound" that "carried farther than its English equivalent," an important consideration in such a large geographic space as Australia. Cooee did not invite cross cultural bonding – although it had the potential to do so since Europeans were plainly mimicking Aborigines. Instead, the European adoption of Cooee, their appropriation of a sound, distanced the two groups. Moreover, Europeans in Australia exaggerated the extent to which the sound was a generalized Aboriginal sound and term (chances are it was limited to a few Aboriginal groups but not shared by others until Europeans spread the sound to them) in an effort to authenticate themselves. Cooee did not bring colonizers and colonized closer "but, as a term of exclusively local origin, it served to bind the *colonists* together." Cooee became the sound of Australian identity. The Aboriginal sound had become white Australia's "call of the bush." It was a sound that allowed Australians to construct their identity at home and abroad, to identify who was genuinely Australian and who was a newcomer by the authenticity of the sound. In this way, white Australians appropriated and then incorporated an Aboriginal sound to form part of their own national identity.[36]

Hearing, listening, sounds, noises, aurality generally, were not simply peripheral to modernity, existing on the outskirts, but, rather, deeply implicated in its daily elaboration. Hearing had occupied an important post in the ancient and medieval world, where it was considered a reliable sense, a sentinel of sorts, a sense that could reveal truth and had a meaningful intellectual component. The print revolution, the Renaissance, the Enlightenment, all enthusiastically promoted the power of the eye, but hearing seemed to hold its own, with no discernible dilution of its social and intellectual importance. In fact, hearing, sound, and aurality generally were critical in many ways to the unfolding of modernity and to downplay its importance only deafens us to the meaning and trajectory of key developments of the post-Enlightenment era.

3

Smelling

Creating a Stink

Historical writing on the history of smell, measured by quantity, has some way to go before it catches up with that on hearing. Given the importance of scent and smell to any number of societies throughout history, the absence of monographs dealing with the topic in any sustained manner is curious. Over a decade ago in their pioneering study, *Aroma: The Cultural History of Smell*, Constance Classen, David Howes, and Anthony Synnott observed: "Odours form the building blocks of cosmologies, class hierarchies and political orders; they can enforce social structures or transgress them... But smell is repressed in the modern West, and its social history ignored."[1] While the work that has been done on the history of smell since is generally of a high quality and while the history of smell and olfaction is beginning to generate sustained interest among historians, we still await full-length treatments of the history of smell for any number of times and places.

We have, though, just about enough work on the topic to know that if hearing remained important during and after the print revolution and if aurality was important to the evolution of modernity and European colonial adventures, the same was equally true with regard to smell. Important during antiquity for a number of reasons, olfaction retained its currency during and after the Enlightenment, especially in the context of colonization and the establishment of systems of unfree labor and racial and class exploitation. Smell, more than any other sense perhaps, served to create and mark the "other," at once justifying various forms of subjugation and serving as a barrier against meaningful integration into host or dominant societies.

Beyond smell's consistently classificatory function, there were important shifts in the role and meaning of smell. Premodern Westerners understood smell to have special spiritual significance and tied it closely to physical health. Smell also indicated truth and was a sense associated with knowledge. While modernity reconfigured scent, sometimes downplaying it in favor of vision, smelling remained critical as authenticator of socially generated and politically motivated "truths." Olfactory shifts, the emergence of new scents, and the push to deodorize did not necessarily mean that smell became less important with modernity. Victorian literature, for example, was full of commentary on smells, their absence, their desirability, frequently couched in an apologetic nostalgia for scents lost courtesy of the industrial revolution. Nostalgic smells stood for tradition, substance, essence, meaning, and their continued popularity in the Victorian mind meant that, symbolically and metaphorically, scents remained authoritative and deeply implicated in iterations of class, gender, race, and ethnicity in twentieth-century conversations about who smelled and why.[2]

Smellscapes of the Ancient and Medieval West

Scents were extremely important to antiquity. Smells, after all, transcended private and public in the ancient world. In Greece, for example, perfumes and oils smelling of thyme, mint, marjoram, and palm coated the body, scenting it for both personal and public olfactory consumption. Scents also infused communal dinners, roses often doing the work, as was also the case with the Romans. Scent was used widely in the ancient world at group gatherings and sporting events – spectators at games held in Syria, for example, were anointed with perfumes as they entered the stadium. This collective olfactory practice stands in contrast to the modern use of highly individuated perfumes intended for largely personal use or application. Other evidence points to the use of smell to effect social designation. Socrates, for example, maintained that slaves and free men had different odors and worried that the widespread use of perfume might mask the distinction.[3]

Olfaction was also linked to ideas concerning physical health. Smells pointed to the cause of a disease and indicated symptoms: pungent and fragrant odors were understood to ward off diseases, themselves believed to be carried by smells. Galen, the ancient Greek physician, while emphasizing consultation with patients, recognized the importance of the physician's sense of smell in diagnosing disease. The nose could detect odors from the patient, especially from the breath. In ancient medicine, then, the nose was not simply a reliable sense: it was the sense that could detect at a depth and level beyond the eye. While the physician's eyes were limited to scouring the surface of the patient's body, his nose could excavate clues and penetrate beyond the skin and surface to achieve a deeper, more meaningful diagnosis.[4]

The Romans, according to Béatrice Caseau's detailed work on olfaction in the ancient world, suppressed bodily odors with perfume and went so far as to define space by deploying different smells. Different odors marked public spaces and celebrations, religious events, and individual rooms within the home. Smell helped define space because each space functioned in a specific way and often served to unite the corporeal world with the spiritual. Scents were often understood by the Romans to serve as especially useful and effective conduits between the two worlds. Smell was so important to Roman thinking that the trade in spices, aromatics, and incense was both geographically expansive – even the smaller urban centers traded Indian spices – and financially extensive.[5]

But it was in the realm of religion that smell, scents, and olfaction reigned in the ancient world. Broadly understood, "Incense, traveling through the air, was believed to attract and unite humans and gods, while the absence of odour, or unpleasant odours, had the opposite effect." In ancient Greek mythology, the very soul was understood as a perfume of sorts because it was associated with breath. Obedience to YHWH made humanity smell sweet to the Lord's nose and the Hebrew Bible is replete with references to scent, sacrifice, and aroma's relationship to knowledge and truth. The book of Tobit (third century BCE) contains references to smell and spirituality and the notion that sanctity had a distinctively sweet odor was widespread. As Ian D. Ritchie has shown, the odor of a right sacrifice reached God's nostrils but a wrong sacrifice was always sniffed out and God could be irritated by misleading sacrificial odors as much as he was pleased by right ones. God's nose, then, could detect truth through smell and it was this association between knowledge and olfaction that probably made aroma such an important part of worship in the Hebraic tradition. For example, the incense burned "as a symbol of the prayers of the people to Yahweh in the liturgy of ancient Israel was made to the special formula found in Exod. 30.34–38," which was not to be used for any other function and was set apart for the Tabernacle service only. Ibn Ezra, the medieval Jewish theologian, reckoned smell more reliable than sight when divining an individual's religious virtues. Sin stank while the presence of the Holy Spirit emitted a sweet odor. On the whole, smell played an important part in Hebraic theology and practice, meditated between spirit and body, and infused daily ritual.[6]

Scent and smells were also critical to early Christianity. While some evidence suggests that early Christians rejected incense and perfumes because of their association with what they understood as pagan rituals and their supposed ability to induce indolence and pleasure, such an emphasis incorrectly dilutes the importance of smell and olfaction to early Christians. In daily Christian life, for example, scents were considered appropriate and proper in terms of grooming and, in the fourth century, when Constantine adorned the Roman basilicas with "golden censers," the importance of smell and incense was "openly admitted" in the Christian Church. Given the importance of smell to adjudicating good and bad, sin and holiness, paradise and hell in early Christian theology, the open embrace of smell and olfaction as a part of the Christian practice is hardly surprising.[7]

The Syrian theologian, St. Ephrem (c. 306–73 BCE), for example, used olfactory images and motifs to frame what he understood as a "basic human experience of smell" and how it revealed knowledge of God. Ephrem had little interest in establishing a mind/body dichotomy, preferring instead to show how knowledge of God was at once cognitive and sensory. He understood the "fragrance of life" to reveal truth about both bodily and spiritual knowing. This idea was premised on the belief that the Christian God was one of revelation – who revealed himself in every place and to humans via their senses. In other words, Ephrem gave the sense of smell its due place, alongside the usually favored senses of sight and sound. Joining images of Christ as Word and Light were motifs associating Christ with a "Glorious Lilly" and a "Treasure of Perfumes" which meant that the act of inhaling the scent of Christ was not only possible but itself an act of divine encounter. In other words, Ephrem articulated an argument that helped Christianity embrace scent. "From its inception until late in the fourth century," argues Susan Ashbrook Harvey, "Christianity had excluded incense from its worship and devotional practices, the only religion of the ancient Mediterranean world to do so," partly in an effort to distinguish themselves from pagans and Jews. Ephrem rejected the pagan use of olfaction as false but found worth in Jewish practice. For Ephrem, scent and incense operated to unite sacrifice and knowledge for, like martyrs, incenses were cast into fires, their scents rising up and established the connection from the physical to the divine.[8]

Early Christians, according to other interpretations, certainly reacted against the use of scent and unguents apparent in Roman and Greek religion and mythology by, for example, banning the use of perfumes "because of their associations with Roman 'idolatry', and their assumed tendency to lead to sensualism." But olfactory suppression and policing was not straightforward. By the mid-fifth century, Christianity had reconstituted the meaning of smells and their religious significance so that they took on meanings beyond sensuality and paganism. Priests were believed to smell sweet, in effect disseminating what Paul called "the aroma of Christ." Perhaps not coincidentally, the first rosaries were likely made of dried rose petals. The Crusades further heightened the European taste for strong scents. Eastern spices and perfumes especially made their way into medieval life and helped give a profoundly olfactory dimension to ideas about the nature – and scent – of the afterlife.[9]

Whatever the specifics concerning early Christian rejection or embrace of scent, it remains clear that for much of the ancient world, when it came to expressions and practice of religious faith especially, smell operated in tandem and enjoyed a rough equality with hearing and seeing and, at times, it trumped both.

Smells Modern: Scent at the Great Divide

There is no doubt that modernity helped deaden smell in favor of sight, as Constance Classen's brilliant history of the rose makes clear. Before the Enlightenment, the rose in early modern Western Europe was thoroughly olfactory in its social importance, its scent embedded in ancient ideas relating to spiritual truth and bodily health. Cherished not only for its esthetic value, the rose in pre-Enlightenment Europe was prized for its scent because of the values associated with its smell. According to Classen, the Enlightenment invested much greater authority in how roses looked, and florists started to cultivate the flower for its visual esthetic, not its scent. Because the Enlightenment devalued the old symbolic importance of scent and elevated the importance of the eye as the sense of truth, the scent of the rose became increasingly subordinated to the way it looked.[10]

That much said, "The sixteenth century's increased sensitivity to visual beauty," notes Classen, "was accompanied by an increased sensitivity to olfactory beauty." English gardens were intended to please the eye – topiary and geometric designs featured prominently – but they also catered to the nose with specific flowers placed strategically for their olfactory pleasure, as Francis Bacon described at some length in 1625. True, powerful forces worked actively to lessen the salience of smell in early modern Europe. The Protestant Reformation, for example, "led to the discrediting of miraculous proofs of holiness such as the odour of sanctity, the prohibition of incense in Protestant churches, and to a disapprobation of olfactory (and other) sensuality." Some radical Protestants, the Puritans especially, were fiercely dismissive of perfumes and musk, believing them to darken and cloud the spirit and inspire sin rather than facilitate communion with God.[11]

Yet no process sweeps clean and olfaction found resuscitation in the hands of the Jesuits and the Catholic Reformation, at least in Germany. Although German Catholicism was extremely fractured in the 1550s, courtesy of the immense success of Luther, Calvin, Zwingli, and others, it began to revive in the 1560s and 1570s not least because of the activities of the Society of Jesus, the Jesuits, and their emphasis on the sensory experience of Catholicism. Ignatius of Loyola (c.1491–1556) did much to lay the groundwork and explicate the role not just of vision but of the other senses, and especially smell, in shaping the Jesuits' message. In *The Spiritual Exercises*, first published in Rome in 1548, Ignatius established the framework directing Jesuit behavior and beliefs and the senses occupied critical ground. According to Jeffrey Chipps Smith, "Ignatius was first and foremost a sensualist, in that he clearly recognized that one should utilize all of one's capabilities when attempting to understand God." Sight was important, of course, and he recommended the creation of mental pictures in the course of spiritual contemplation. But the other senses were very important in, for example, inspiring genuine understanding of hell, something that demanded that one "smell with the smell of smoke, sulphur, dregs and putrid things." Taste, touch, and hearing also had roles to play but Ignatius seemed especially interested in the senses of smell and taste in animating memory and facilitating communion with God. Hearing, he argued, was the sense of faith, insight into faith empowered sight, touch derived from the union of love, from the joy of love came the power to taste, and from hope was derived the power to smell. God's grace empowered the individual's spiritual senses and allowed man to experience the presence of God. Ignatius urged one to "smell and to taste ... the infinite fragrance and sweetness of the Divinity, of the soul, and of its virtues." These were not abstractions but, rather, clues to finding God's presence in daily life. God could be detected in the scent of a flower, for example, and smells offered Christians a highly personal way to communicate with God. This helps explain why, for example, Michel de Montaigne in 1580 commented on the continued use of incense in churches, a practice he considered "so ancient and widespread" that it had assumed a universal quality allowing for spiritual contemplation. In other words, even as ascetic Protestant forces (themselves easily exaggerated) were gaining ground, the Jesuits kept alive – in powerful and persistent ways – the role of the senses in religious thought and daily experience.[12]

Similarly, if more secularly, concerns about smell and olfaction were very much at the forefront of social policy in, for example, sixteenth- and seventeenth-century English cities. London's mayors and aldermen, writes Mark S. R. Jenner, "were preoccupied with the extirpation of stench and noisome air." The association of smell and disease led to a number of orders for cleaning the streets of smells and odors. In 1631, officials in York urged people to soak sponges with white wine vinegar and camphor to ward off the plague; all infected dwellings were to be perfumed with rosemary, bay, and juniper. Smell occupied such an important place in municipal and social policy because odors were understood to affect and penetrate the body directly and, especially, the brain, an idea inherited from Galen, endorsed by the Arabian physician and philosopher, Abu Ali al-Husain ibn Abdallah ibn Sina, or Avicenna (980–1037), and generally agreed upon by sixteenth-century Western medical authorities. Seventeenth-century medical opinion tended to reject this thinking and stressed instead the effect of smell on nerves, although authorities continued to debate whether or not smells themselves were physical entities taken into the body or immaterial wafts that were detectable primarily by the brain and mind. Medical ideas about smell, then, circulated in important and meaningful ways and they came to shape and inform public health regulations in early modern English towns in the same period that witnessed the empowerment of vision and seeing.[13]

Others, Smells, and Selves in the Modern World

Modernity was deeply indebted to smell and olfaction. Smell not only helped elaborate a number of key modern developments – industrialization, the construction of class identity, ideas of selfhood and otherness, imperial and colonial ventures, elaborations of gender and race, to note just a few – but it is difficult to appreciate the full extent and nature of these developments without attending to the history of smell and smelling.

Constance Classen maintains, quite correctly, that "The ocular obsession of Enlightenment thought did not completely oust smell from the cultural arena, however, for perfumes continued to be extensively used through this period." Olfactory codes played key classificatory roles, especially when it came to gender. If post-Enlightenment men were increasingly associated with the sense of sight, truth, intellect, and knowledge, women were increasingly indexed to one (or more) olfactory categories – the spicy signature of the hyper-sexualized woman, the stench of socially marginal women (prostitutes, for example; *puta* in Spanish means whore, derived from the Latin word for putrid), and the perfumed, fragrant, often floral, clean scent of ideal womanhood. Men, perceived as champions of the new industrial, capitalist, and visualist order, were understood in late nineteenth-century Britain to function largely as eye-men, surveying the world, viewing empires, scanning horizons. Women, conversely, were custodians of smells, especially domestic ones, and particularly smells that accorded with their supposedly more emotional and intuitive nature.[14]

Class distinctions – subjective and objective – so very constitutive of modernity, were also indebted to olfaction. English elites were especially adept at demarcating class through the nose. They, of course, inhabited largely inodorate or especially fragrant places, their own bodies manifestly delightful to any nose; by contrast, the English working class stank – its putrid wretches consigned to reeking environments and tenements which even their extravagant, clumsy use of coarse perfumes could never truly mask. George Orwell expressed this powerful conceit pithily in the 1930s. The "secret of class distinctions in the West," he remarked, can be summarized in "four frightful words… *The lower classes smell.*" Workers could put up with their own stench, so the argument went, because they had such dulled nostrils; elites, by contrast, possessed heightened olfactory sensitivities. That animals were often assumed to possess such heightened sensitivity to smell went without much comment.[15]

The odor of class – and the class of odor – started to become especially important in the mid-eighteenth century when Western elites increasingly sought to suppress and deny odor. By some estimations, this amounted to nothing short of an "olfactive revolution." An idea championed initially by nobles and aristocrats but quickly embraced by the emerging middle class in the nineteenth century, olfaction increasingly took on class importance with urbanization and industrialization. Who was deemed smelly and who was considered inodorate – and who got to define the meaning and value of various scents – was critical for class formation which, in turn, was linked to ideas about selfhood. As the nineteenth-century Western bourgeoisie started to stamp the laboring classes especially as reeking, they also paraded themselves as largely inodorate, lacking in bad scent and, in the process, they heightened consciousness not just of class smells but individuated smells. Consciousness of how one smelled as an individual enabled the construction of olfactory others.[16]

A good example of how this larger process played out is apparent in *The Foul and the Fragrant: Odor and the French Social Imagination*, Alain Corbin's wonderful analysis of the changing perceptions of the French, 1750–1880, toward smells. Unlike some early historians, including Lucien Febvre who claimed that people had gradually lost their sense of smell in the sixteenth century, Corbin shows that olfaction was very much alive between 1750 and 1850. Corbin examined the creation of social and physical distance between "dangerous" smells/smelling people, the arrangement of public and private spaces, and the trumpeting of class authority reflected in the bourgeois control of the sense of smell to score social others, usually the criminal and working poor. Although he perhaps discounted the importance of science in redefining why certain smells became increasingly understood as not indicative of disease (David S. Barnes's recent study does an admirable job of explaining how the scientific discovery of germ theory in late nineteenth-century France served to disassociate smells and the idea of disease), Corbin nevertheless offered a powerful class analysis to consider the impact of smelling on notions of the self. The arrangement of private space and the use of personal, often individuated fragrances entailed delimiting and isolating odors and so inaugurated among individuals a new encounter with their own body and even a new narcissism.[17]

"The terror inspired by putrid diseases and the miasmas which propagated them," remarks Corbin with regard to post-Revolutionary France, encouraged an "olfactory vigilance which was always on the lookout for threatening putrefaction." Smells in overcrowded urban areas – excrement, stench from industry, the reek of animal products – gave rise to a heightened sensitivity to smell and led to strident efforts to stamp stench out through legislation and the regulation of industrial "nuisances," themselves "part of that wider programme of control and surveillance which has been revealed by Michel Foucault." The idea that smell and disease were closely associated, one so popular during the Middle Ages and earlier, had not disappeared by the nineteenth century.[18]

Up until the 1840s, French urban municipalities and councils tolerated smells generated by new industries, especially those using chemicals and putrid products. Initial complaints quickly lapsed into "resignation and tacit acceptance" by authorities. There was also an important class dynamic at work: officials entrusted to regulate smelly industries found that workers inside chemical buildings seemed unbothered by the smells and pollution. Worker habituation suggested something about the insensitivity of proletarian noses. In this respect, workers did not have heightened senses associated with animals but they did have deadened senses increasingly associated with, well, proletarians. The dullness of the peasant and worker nose, their olfactory insensibility to stench and the dangers associated with smells, helped generate bourgeois stereotypes linking poverty and disease, manual labor and dirt, and a general doltish proletarian sensibility that proved remarkably enduring and a handy justification for the population of slums by people who, apparently (and conveniently, for elites) did not know the difference between stench and (good) perfume anyway.[19]

Interestingly enough, complaints in Paris about the increasing use of stench-producing technologies (coal, bitumen, rubber factories) in the 1840s were generated less because of their effect on the nose but more because of their effect on the eyes – a point that tends to support claims about the emergence of vision as the sense most in need of protection. As Corbin put it, smoke was a preoccupation less because it stank but more because it was "blackish and opaque, attacked the lungs, dirtied facades and darkened the atmosphere just when people were beginning to develop a concern for light."[20]

Legal definitions of what was stench and what was not were slower to evolve than casual, daily definitions, which seemed to circulate with frightening ease. Between 1840 and 1864, for example, American courts adjudicated differently on industries that emitted stench and noise depending not on the specifics of the senses but, rather, whether the sensory nuisance was rooted in a deep historical past (especially if grounded in English common law) or associated with a new industry. Traditional nuisances were inherited from the Middle Ages, elaborated during the colonial period, and still existed in modernizing, nineteenth-century America. A body of law had established that the scent from animal urine, blood, offal and the smells produced as a result of boiling organic materials were material nuisances. Colonial governments, for example, required offenders to clean slaughterhouses and forbade them to throw waste into the streets. On occasion, they even made them relocate their businesses. The same type of adjudication continued into the early nineteenth century when applied against these "traditional" industries. The guiding belief here was that "people had a right to live in and travel through neighborhoods where their noses would not be assaulted by terrible smells that might carry disease, even death." But smells and fumes, even if actually toxic, produced by newer industries, those associated with the industrial revolution – textile mills, smelters, mines, steam-powered industries, railroads – remained unopposed by the courts because it was difficult to persuade judges and juries that the sensory effects of the new industries were, in fact, as damaging as those produced by the old ones. "Proof" was difficult to come by when tagging a new industry as dangerous whereas the old threats had such a genealogy as to constitute prima facie presumptive nuisances. Moreover, judges did not have a cultural context with which to label and understand the new emissions as especially offensive or dangerous and it took them until after the Civil War and into the twentieth century to conceptualize the new noises and the new smells produced by new industries as, in fact, presumptive nuisances. The U.S. legal system took time to define what was sensorially offensive and what was not.[21]

Ideas of progress, of civilization, were closely indexed to ideas concerning smell and class elsewhere in the world, especially in those New World societies heavily colonized by Europeans. Take, for example, an important aspect of the history of olfaction in nineteenth- and early twentieth-century Chile. Private and state-sponsored efforts to modernize Valparaiso, for example, included beliefs about how a modern city should smell and how best to go about controlling its smellscape. Beginning in the 1870s, Valparaiso's city council commissioned the design and building of a sewer system in an effort to improve and modernize the city. Modernization in this context meant trying to contain and eradicate the seasonal stench emitted from streams that ran near the city and the open sewage that sometimes coursed through its streets. By the early 1880s, a rudimentary sewage system was in place but the stench remained and complaints grew. Newspaper editorial reports compared Valparaiso's "smelly sewers with those of other cities," including Paris and Calcutta. Officials deemed the Chilean city's stench injurious to health and blamed the sewer system. Unless every neighborhood were tied in to the system, some municipal officials argued, a partial network could not safely contain the sewage and the smell. In the early 1880s, the city's poor neighborhoods remained outside the system and tended to use streams and outhouses to dispose of refuse. In other words, officials argued that the sewage system would work only if the poor were required to connect to it. In this way, bad smell and its perceived threat to public health seems to have centered upon the lower classes in Valparaiso, just as it did in Rio de Janeiro, Paris, and elsewhere.[22]

The use of olfactory stereotypes to "other" was hardly limited to the West and its colonies. Judging by admittedly limited evidence, olfactory stereotypes also informed urban–rural distinctions in China in the 1930s. City dwellers in southern Chinese cities associated country folk with the smell of garlic and tended to believe the scent typical of northern peasants. To the Chinese farmer, garlic was the signature smell of home and working with the land; to the Chinese urbanite in the 1930s, it was the mark of inferiority, something to be avoided and ridiculed.[23]

If smell was deployed to delineate gender, class, and, as in the Chinese example, urban and rural distinctions, it should come as no surprise that it also informed in very powerful ways constructions of race and the language and politics of racism. If the Chinese in China during the 1930s used smell to categorize one another, a similar process worked against Chinese immigrants in the United States. In the late nineteenth and early twentieth century in California, odor became a topic of intense debate. As Connie Y. Chiang has shown, two "odor conflicts" unfolded in Monterey in the 1890s and again a few decades later. The first conflict concerned Chinese fishermen whose habit of laying out their squid to dry offended local white residents and tourists, especially those in the Hotel Del Monte. White Americans believed the squid – and, increasingly by association, the Chinese men who caught it – reeked and attached the smell to prevailing ideas about inferiority, lack of cleanliness, and difference. Those attempting to promote tourism characterized the Chinese fishing villages as "unspeakably dirty and redolent with the odor of decaying fish." The Pacific Improvement Company, as owner of both the hotel and the Chinese fishing village, was the arbiter in the case and ended up siding with Monterey's white residents and, in effect, endorsed their claims about who smelled and why. The company, Chiang shows, "used odors to leverage its political influence and create an excuse for removing the Chinese and sanitizing the shoreline."[24]

Odor conflict again erupted in the 1930s. This time, the producers of odor, so it was claimed, were not the Chinese but, rather, the sardine cannery factories along Ocean View Avenue. The smells from so-called Cannery Row were so great that the city had come to be known as Monterey-by-the-Smell. By the 1930s, real estate developers and hotel owners, along with tourist-friendly politicians and again led by the Hotel Del Monte, initiated a legal battle to suppress the stench. Unlike the 1890s, though, the fish industry prevailed not least because they made a more powerful economic argument than that offered by the tourist industry. The sardine industry did not deny that it produced a smell but it did claim that tourists' noses were overly sensitive and that to eliminate the fishy odor would be an economic blow to the area, especially for working families in a time of pronounced economic recession. The association of race and smell in the first instance enabled the tourist industry to triumph, not least because the end of the nineteenth century was a period keenly interested in race and America's future prosperity and how immigrants might threaten that security. In the 1930s, the prospect for economic development prevailed over the tourist industry. In both instances, smells produced visceral reactions on all sides. Moreover, because, as Chiang argues, "odors were subjective" and defied easy measurement, what smelled and who smelled was defined principally through the skein of power relations, established not by some objective standard but, rather, by those who held the greatest social, political, and economic power.[25]

Elsewhere in the New World and in wholly undemocratic social systems – for example in slave-based nineteenth century Rio de Janeiro – unfree labor was used by elites to protect themselves from what they perceived as the smell of the lower orders. In Rio, slavery acted as a gatekeeper, distancing elites from the odor of lower classes. Over the course of the nineteenth century, "slum dwellers, not the slums, became the agents of disease" for Brazilian elites. "The poor and their teeming slums had once belonged to the world of the street, the world kept at a distance by residents able to screen out the filth, smells, or noise with their walled gardens and shuttered windows and who relied on their servants as go-betweens, able to preserve the illusion of their own safekeeping." But in the last decades of the century, Rio's slaveholders increasingly had to rely less on the crumbling regime of slavery and more on hired workers that lived in the lower-class slums, the *corticos*, and were believed to carry their poor hygiene and disease into the elite household. The perceived smell of the *corticos* put elites in a dilemma: they needed labor but feared the smell of the laborer. Because laundresses washed their clothes, because some elites believed "'bad smell' came from the 'infected matter in the dirty clothes,'" elites fretted about the possibility of contamination. Hiring wet-nurses proved similarly problematic: prescriptive literature often suggested choosing a safe wet-nurse on the basis of visuality – the shade of her skin color – but, increasingly, smell became important as well: their milk should be "odorless." With the collapse of slavery, the possibility of creating a household secure against the sensory disorder of the streets became increasingly challenging for elites in Rio de Janeiro.[26]

So too – and even more obviously – with whites in the southern United States, many of whom justified twentieth-century segregation on the basis that African Americans had an innate odor, one they associated with filth and disease. Smell was used to justify separating bodies black and white in public space. Contradictions and tensions abounded in the creation and elaboration of this particular sensory stereotype. First, the argument that blacks smelled to white noses should have posed some troubling worries to whites who argued that they, by nose alone, could detect racial difference. After all, suggested one nineteenth-century writer, modern man's senses had been dulled and "contaminated with the smells of perfumery, distilleries, chemical works, and vile cooking." Only "savage tribes" had a heightened sense of smell, one "almost as acute as in lower mammalia." Peruvian Indians, for example, "can distinguish the different races, whether European, American Indian, or Negro, by the sense of smell alone." What, then, are we to make of "civilized" white southerners who claimed they could smell blackness? The contradiction was elided, the sensory construction of racial difference having by this time taken on an ineluctable and unquestioned logic of its own.[27]

Second, many whites in the American South, just like Brazilian slaveholders, contravened their own injunctions on a daily basis by using black labor in their homes, thus engaging in private what they demarcated in public. Whites offered some convoluted arguments in response – that their maids and domestic help were not as odor-ridden as the rest of the black population, for example – but, fundamentally, they relied on what they considered the emotive power of smell in order to avoid engaging in an argument about the logic of their sensory stereotype. Whites held the subjective authority to define blackness as reeking and they appealed to the viscerality of the stereotype to foreclose sustained conversations that might have interrogated their logic's integrity.[28] The only intellectual critique of the olfactory stereotype came, in fact, from African Americans. Southern blacks maintained that their scent was the product simply of wretched living conditions, of environment, rather than inherent. Here, it was left up to dispossessed blacks and lower orders to ask the hard, materialist questions about an easy and thoughtless olfactory stereotype. Unlike some workers who came to believe the stereotypes elites leveled against them, southern blacks challenged them, not by inverting them – they rarely argued that elite southern whites stank – but, rather, by testing the basis of the white argument and, in the process, exposing it for the emotional, illogical non-sense it was.[29]

The racial olfactory conceits that informed modern segregation in the American South also gave shape to European colonial projects in modern Africa. White charges of black stench in twentieth-century Zimbabwe, and southern Africa generally, were repeated with an intensity and frequency that white southerners would have found reassuring. Like whites in the American South, white Rhodesians rarely specified what they thought Africans smelled like. The emotional and subjective power of the charge actually precluded that sort of detail lest it invite serious investigation of the stereotype itself. And, just like southern whites and Brazilian slaveholders, Rhodesians happily used black domestic labor even as they leveled the charge of stench, lack of hygiene, and possible disease. Remarkably, they eagerly advocated that Africans use soap while they argued, simultaneously, that their odor was innate. Whatever the contradictions of white ideology, they were more than sufficient to establish a colonial, segregated society.[30]

Lastly, it should come as no surprise that olfactory othering extended to ethnicity and nationality and was used to denigrate outsiders and, simultaneously, bolster and give shape to emerging national and ethnic identities. Like Western Europeans and Americans, Russians, for example, used smell to define otherness within their own society. In the late 1920s, Russian railroad workers frequently claimed that Kazakhs, with whom they labored on a daily basis, stank. The charge was one way in which native Russians marked ethnicity and race.[31] In a more nationalist vein, in the Cold War period of the 1940s the Russians liked to distinguish themselves from the capitalist Americans on the basis of scent; Communist Soviets and ethnic Russians – the two seemed to blend – understood themselves as living in a vibrant, full-textured olfactory world where "everything smells," while in contrast Americans suffered under a "bland sterile air" in their homes. Here, American air-conditioning, the circulation of air, seemed to be the culprit; Russians preferred their air-tight homes, windows puttied shut in winter, the door the only vent, "so the smells remain in homes, whether they are city homes or peasant huts." Russians also "expect things to smell, especially food," and they believed that American fruits and vegetables were worryingly odorless. In other words, Russians styled their smellscape as richer, fuller, more emotional and sensuous than the tepid, faint, and withered American one. Communism was, by extension, more sensorially robust, even more honest, more attached to nature, the product of more authentic and real smells and inhabited by people with stronger noses. American and, by implication, capitalist olfaction, was abstracted, consumed, unauthentic, and divorced from lived experience. Interestingly, this extended to stores, too. Even though American supermarkets and department stores were busily infusing their stores with artificial sensory delights – lighting, music, and smells – in the 1950s, their effect paled when compared to what appears to have been untouched, "real" smells in Russian stores. In the United States "one can walk from one floor of a department store to another, without being able to tell by smell what merchandise is being sold. In Russia every store smelled of its wares, and smelled strongly."[32]

Perceptions, stereotypes, and actual smells circulated in both the ancient and modern worlds with at once intense intimacy and broad applicability. Smells were simultaneously individuated and personal and also used to delineate any number of groups, races, genders, classes, ethnicities, and nationalities. Although we are in dire need of detailed studies for both the West and non-West that help us understand how, precisely, olfactory protocols and meanings migrated from antiquity, through the Middle Ages, and into modernity, we have enough work to suggest that such a migration did occur, that the history of olfaction and the ways that smells were used in many regions of the ancient and modern world experienced a striking continuity, at least insofar as olfaction and scent was believed to be an authenticator of truth, a source of knowledge, and, in some cases, a reliable indicator of the true state of faith and a sense that could be reliably invoked to shape social relations, difference, and ideas of self and national identity.

4

Tasting

A good deal of what we know about the history of taste is courtesy of philosophers, some literary scholars, and work on the history of individual foods, especially in the ways in which they functioned as commodities. Thanks principally to anthropologists whose interest in the topic blossomed beginning mainly in the 1970s, the history of taste, at least as it is framed and understood by the history of food, drink, and cuisine, has quite a deep genealogy. In fact, Carolyn Korsmeyer describes work on "Gustation in History" as "probably the largest field of study for taste, food, and eating habits," with historically minded anthropologists still at the vanguard of the historical study of taste and how it informed the emergence of class identity, ideas about gender and race, esthetic taste and judgment, the meaning of modernity and, perhaps most obviously and enduringly, how taste functioned to give deep, sometimes emotional, meaning to modern ideas concerning ethnic and national identity.[1]

(Re)Pasts in the Ancient and Early Modern World

Eating and drinking functioned in a number of ways in the ancient world. Public displays of consumption often had legal force, for example. Drinking a toast in public marked legal transactions in Homeric Greece and, in the ancient Near East, tasting, eating, and drinking also communicated "a legal transaction or event to immediate parties or to witnesses." Less publicly, medical diagnosis in ancient Greece relied on taste to some extent. According to Galen, a patient's sweat should be tasted, the physician's tongue ascertaining its saltiness or acridity. Much could be learned: bitter tasting sweat hinted at jaundice, for example. Taste also held important religious and spiritual implications.

A Hebrew tradition held "the Old Covenant with Yahweh was a meal taken together in his presence." Likewise, eating unleavened bread at Passover was a sign to Moses from God "that the law of God may be in your mouth."[2]

More telling, taste and gustation helped arrange social authority. As Carolyn Korsmeyer has made clear, the sense of taste, at least for some key ancient philosophers, was ascribed a status as a lower, bodily, less intellectual sense than sight. Plato and Aristotle lumped taste with the supposedly proximate senses of touch and smell while touting seeing and hearing as the only genuinely philosophical and distinctly "masculine" senses. Greek philosophy generally, shows Korsmeyer, associated the senses of truth, steady reason, and knowledge with men and paired women and the lower senses, thus reinforcing assumptions – popular then and, as Korsmeyer suggests, now – about women's supposed indifference to philosophy and preoccupation with gustation, olfaction, and tactility, senses most closely associated with food and sex. Although Plato was not entirely clear why vision especially supposedly fostered wisdom and philosophy, it may be that he understood sight as less connected to, and in more distant service to, the bodily senses and their supposed pull on the appetite. Aristotle was clearer about why taste ranked low on the sensory scale. While he acknowledged that taste was not necessarily simply sybaritic and without reflection – for example, he noted, that while animals eat, only humans taste and have the ability to savor (to think about) their food – he observed that taste and touch were the two senses most associated with pleasure and pain and it was that engagement with the body that threatened to overwhelm intellect. Food's function as the source of health and life was, on one level, innocent. In another respect, though, the taste of food could carry the sense beyond the merely functional into sensory and bodily indulgence. Taste always had to be disciplined against over-indulgence – a particular challenge, since tasting was a necessary function of life and always prone to lead the individual towards gluttony. In this context, argues Korsmeyer, Aristotle injected a gendered reading of the senses which doubted the reliability of women's sight – thus distancing them from what he considered the highest and most intellectual sense – and implied that women were more susceptible to the baser, more emotional lure of appetite and taste.[3]

The discriminatory and classificatory function of taste and consumption in Greek life is not especially surprising given the central role food played in Greek mythology. Foodstuffs and meals helped elaborate hierarchy outside of human relations and in Greek cosmology generally.

The sacrificial meal, for example, separated man from beast. While both humans and animals were understood to need food to survive, only the food of man – and woman – had been cultivated, grown (especially cereals), and cooked, while animals, with their less refined sense of taste, consumed food that was raw and commensurate with their inability to taste. But humans were not gods and the sacrificial meal, while serving as the channel of communication between earth and heaven, distinguished the two. While man's share "of the sacrificed animal is the dead, corruptible meat: the gods' share is the smoke from the charred bones, the smell of perfumes, and incorruptible spices." Men tasted, gods smelled, and the sacrificial meal served to subordinate taste to smell and locate man beneath the gods. In this, and other ways, taste not only helped frame gender in Greek society but functioned as a sense that differentiated man from animals and man from the gods.[4]

The discriminating function of food and taste was not limited to ancient Greece. Food and power was connected in ancient Rome where the "gastronomic pretensions" of the elite resulted in a number of sumptuary laws designed to "control the expenditure on food and to limit the extent of conspicuous consumption." Neither was the relationship between cuisine, food, and power simply Western. Food was indexed quite precisely to power and hierarchy in diverse non-Western societies, notably those of ancient China, India, and in the Middle East. In China between the seventh and tenth centuries, for example, wine was officially the exclusive preserve of emperors, and Marco Polo commented that the rich ate "the flesh of bigger animals" while the poor consumed "all sorts of unclean flesh." The importation of foreign foods and spices, especially during the Tang dynasty (618–906), further braided the relationship between class and food: rich households relied increasingly on "foreign" food, incorporating spices especially into their tastes, notably Indian-style dishes, while peasant diets remained more conspicuously indigenous and less influenced by "outside" tastes. Moreover, it was during this period that the rich started to manipulate the relationship between time and taste, altering the seasonality of food by using ice as a preservative. Peasants stayed wedded to a more traditional gustatory calendar.[5]

Echoes lingered into the early modern period in the West and elsewhere. An English statute of 1336 – a sumptuary law – limited the number of courses one should consume. The norm was two at each meal, "except on the principal feasts of the year" when "every man may be served with courses at the utmost." Efforts to regulate consumption in this fashion were very much to do not only with religious admonitions against extravagance but class differentiation. In the early modern European context especially, such prohibitions were typical of "the struggle between feudal or quasi-feudal nobilities and urban mercantile bourgeoisies," the former regulating behavior in an effort to shore up class distinctions. And while some evidence suggests that between 1350 and 1550 the diet of the peasantry in Europe was not particularly different to that of the nobility, it seems that such rough gustatory equality (if, in fact, it existed) began to evaporate after around 1600 when a tendency for the rich to eat meat more frequently than the poor became apparent.[6]

Social disciplines concerning food and eating were informed by and reflected in religious dictates. Certainly, early Christianity was not invariably ascetic. On feast days, after all, food and drink were central to Christian forms of celebration. As Anthony Synnott has shown, "sensory gratification could be good, so long as it was directed toward the glory of God" in the early modern period. Some medieval theologians, such as William of Auxerre (c.1150–1231), placed taste firmly within theological and religious discourse. For example, he described "the Eucharist as a mystical feast in which Christ's body and blood are encountered in a spiritually sensuous manner through the soul's spiritual senses." Bread, wine, taste: all served to establish the immediacy and intimacy of Christ's presence. Yet Christians often targeted taste as a sense particularly prone to weakness. Even the sensorially sympathetic Saint Ignatius Loyola, for example, crafted "rules for eating" intended to discipline the sense of taste and lead it away from appetite toward nutrition.[7]

Taste also gave meaning to space and location. Regional cuisines were important to China and remained so, as we will see, well into the twentieth century. Chinese cuisine between the eleventh and thirteenth centuries was often regional, the taste of place holding a great deal of sway over how people understood themselves and their relationship to the larger society. Some of this regionalism was simply a reflection of which foods could be grown where – rice was more available in the South while millet and wheat were grown in the North. More generally, the Chinese did not generally consume milk products simply because the soy bean provided the same sort of nutrition but more economically. But regions also seasoned their cuisines for cultural and historical reasons, a habit usually framed in terms of "tradition" but also subject to the kinds of spices that were available locally. "Traditional" cuisine, the taste of a region, then, was at once cultural and material, influenced by the availability of certain types of food and reflected in the cultural incorporation of those cuisines into local ideas about regional and ethnic fare and taste.⁸

Lastly, as T. Sarah Peterson has shown in her important work, we need to take account of shifts and continuities in taste from the ancient world to the early modern period in the West if we are to understand properly how self-consciously "modern" European ideas about food and taste came into being. The principal change from ancient Greece and Rome, at least in terms of ingredients and food available to (largely elite) palates in thirteenth-century Europe, came about courtesy of Arab and Islamic culinary influence. By way of trade, wars in the sixth century, and territorial aggrandizement in Sicily, the Iberian Peninsula, and areas of the eastern Mediterranean, Arabs brought new tastes to Western Europe. Greatly diminished in importance was honey – the main sweetener in Greece and Rome – and it was replaced by sugar and any number of new spices and coloring agents such as saffron (which imbued food with a visual flavor). By the thirteenth century, these Arabic influences had made their way through the Holy Roman Empire and into Normandy and England, pervading cooking styles and habits throughout Europe during the Middle Ages. Spices smothered food and their relative scarcity served as a way for ruling classes to display and consume their wealth. But food carried baggage and the meaning Islam attached to various foods and their tastes affected the larger political and religious context in which it was consumed. As Peterson explains, while not all Christians viewed "the demands of the body as a hindrance to the soul's quest for God," by the fifth century "the clergy had firmly coalesced around an ideal of sexual continence, and food was linked to desire." Islam, by contrast, contained a different view of the body, paradise, and food. Earthly voluptuous pleasures were to be enjoyed mainly in anticipation of bodily, gustatory ones in celestial paradise. The Islamic admonition to "Eat and drink with relish, for what ye have been doing" traveled widely throughout the Middle Ages and the recipes and foods associated with the belief system were captured in translated Islamic and Arabic manuscript cookbooks that "eschewed the severe ascetic ideal of Christendom in favor of a style of cookery that closely resembled the sensual contemporary Arabic cuisine." Moreover, the Arabic belief in the medical properties of various spices, notably camphor, accorded with medieval European concepts not only of distant geographical paradises but also of divine medicine and were readily assimilated into a worldview that stressed the relationship between astrology, the occult, and food.⁹

Gustation and Modernity

Encounters and Identities

The gustatory link between the ancient world and the early modern and modern West was, in part at least, indebted to political contrivance on the part of some European elites. Again, as Peterson's insightful work shows, the well documented retreat from Arabic and Islamic cuisine in early modern Europe and the subsequent reconstitution of a cuisine that was styled as modern by contemporaries, can be dated to the fifteenth century when "the military threat from the Arab East had become increasingly menacing." The Ottomans claimed Constantinople in 1453 and Turkish forces made headway in the eastern Mediterranean in 1480. Fearful and apprehensive, leading European humanists, such as Aeneas Silvius, Pope Pius II, among others, increasingly sought Europe's "true" historical roots and found their "authentic" heritage in a Greco-Roman past, a largely contrived image of a time and place. Certain types of food and gustatory behaviors – such as the man of culinary taste – were identified with this putatively purer Western heritage and resurrected in an effort to preserve European integrity against Arabic cultural influences in the early modern period. In a very real sense, this usually quite selective appeal to what, for example, the Greeks did with food and said about taste, was an attempt to preserve early modern European culture through food and taste. "In their efforts to revive the sensuality of the ancients," by attending to what they ate, how they ate, and what taste meant, explains Peterson, "the Renaissance humanists," mostly physicians schooled in natural philosophy, "had done the spadework to link the moderns with antiquity."[10]

Beyond this gustatory arc connecting early modern Europe with antiquity, Peterson also shows how taste was deeply implicated in the very heart of the Renaissance and Enlightenment thanks largely to the French. French cuisine in the seventeenth century blended science and sensual motifs, establishing rules and codes for what to eat and how. For example, newly empowered culinary aficionados and literal arbiters of taste deemed sweets suspect not just because they were Arabic, not just because they had not occupied a prominent place in ancient cuisine, but also because they counteracted the appetive powers of salt. French food aimed to stimulate desire and to achieve this fundamental goal they established formal academies for cooking, established rules governing what and how to cook, developed new words for new tastes and foods, and, in the seventeenth century especially, began thinking in terms of food compositions and harmonious structures, thus echoing the larger scientific community's concern with reason, balance, classification, and judgment.[11]

Despite taste's important role in the Enlightenment and scientific discourse, it is nevertheless true that, in some quarters at least, the sense of taste was eclipsed and even captured by sight. Representations of food and associated tastes – gustatory and esthetic – had been popular in Western art since the introduction of the still life genre in the seventeenth century but that association was largely visual and quietly made questions of "taste" abstract and esthetic and divested art of its sensorial quality. Immanuel Kant did much to further the association of sight and taste principally by distinguishing between the faculty of taste – which was an esthetic, transcendent point of view – and the culture of taste, something associated with the tongue, throat, and more animal like. Kant, like others, used one sense – vision – to mask gustation, to describe visual beauty in terms of taste, a sleight of language and hand that, once interrogated, reveals a sensory politics at work. "Vision," explains Jennifer Fisher, "designated taste's name, elides the experience of actual gustatory sensation." Thus, the disinterested Kantian "point of view" reinforced the visuality of art, art best understood from a distance, with perspective, and separate from the observer. It was this masquerading that fed off the Enlightenment empowerment of vision to eclipse taste and wrap esthetics and judgment in visual blankets, divested of gustation.[12]

Not all thinkers, however, held to Kant's perspective. As David Howes and Marc Lalonde compellingly explain, several thinkers, Alexander Pope and David Hume most notably, gave taste "uncharacteristic emphasis in their writings." Such philosophers did not use taste in a simply analogical way (to refer to an esthetic or style) but, rather, referred to taste in a fully textured, thoroughly gustatory manner. Howes and Lalonde ask a fundamental and frequently ignored question: It would, they point out, have been open to these thinkers "to use the time-honored metaphor of the 'inner eye in their discussions of how we discriminate between things and make judgments, but for some reason they preferred to use a gustatory idiom. Why? Why was taste in food so much on the mind of the eighteenth-century thinker? And why did that mind choose taste over sight (or hearing) to evoke its most essential operation – that of *judgment*?" Their answer is that gustatory (and olfactory) discourse increased at precisely the moment when a variety of social boundaries became blurred, smudged, and unstable. Order and the proximate senses, then, were intimately related and this is clear through the history of taste.[13]

Take, for example, that most unlikely of culinary modern nations, England. Various strands of modernity conspired to make mid-eighteenth century English cuisine resolutely bland and uninspiring. It was a cuisine that favored plain meat and potatoes over anything remotely "continental," saucy, or spicy. But what was it that made the English so committed to such fare in the mid-1700s? Howes and Lalonde explain that key aspects of modernity help explain why the English ate what they did and why they liked it. Because food supplies became relatively secure by the 1750s, courtesy of international trade, a stabilizing political order, and economic growth, elites de-emphasized the quantitative consumption of food in favor of a new, qualitative appreciation of food whose supply was steady and reliable. A new conversation, then, evolved concerning food, delicacy, and taste. Connected to this development was the introduction of new foods from abroad – this was, after all, Britain's age of imperial expansion – and a concomitant puffing of nationalism. The discovery of new foods and tastes did not, in the English instance, always lead to a diversification of the diet and the incorporation of different foods (that was many years off); instead, the initial English reaction was to emphasize the Englishness of their national cuisine. In effect, the English wrote nationalism into consumption, foodways, and taste. Food was tied intimately to the emergence of national identity in eighteenth-century Britain and international trade, imperial ambitions, and the workings of political economy cannot be properly understood outside of that process.[14]

In that broad social, political, and economic context emerged an additional meaning, one that made taste an arbiter of class. Unlike ideas of taste nurtured and elaborated during antiquity, which sometimes tended to universalize the idea of taste and equated it with ingestion, digestion, and learning, eighteenth-century philosophical discussions of taste, most notably David Hume's *Of the Standard of Taste* (1757), particularized the idea of taste, marking it as largely subjective, socially delimited, and the provenance of a group of "men of society" who knew good taste and who set themselves up as arbiters of social judgment. In fact, as Howes and Lalonde explain, this recasting of taste was wholly necessary to the new social order of eighteenth-century England and essential if elites were to preserve their cultural authority. Rapidly urbanizing England tended to undermine the authority of the eye. Urbanization, economic modernization, the widespread circulation of cheaper and more accessible visual goods – such as clothes – made it increasingly difficult to see men of true quality. Elites complained bitterly that laborers dressed like gentleman and no amount of sumptuary legislation could stop classes from looking alike. Because vision operated at the surface, its claims to truth were limited to what was exterior. Because the "'truth' of another person's social standing was no longer obvious at first glance", British elites of the eighteenth century – not unlike American ones a century later – became anxious, searching for other ways to locate and fix reality. Enter the sense of taste. Hume, for example, touted taste – an affective, proximate sense – as belonging to elites and known only to elite men, an argument that had an interior and self-fulfilling quality. Because taste was largely subjective it could be owned by a small group and framed in sentimental terms that made it difficult for the laboring classes to emulate. Hume maintained that "a delicacy of taste" helped confine "our choice to a few people ... making us indifferent to the company and conversation of the greater part of men." In place of the feudal order of objective and historically established class distinctions, Hume posited a social order based on subjective, arbitrary sentiment, one mediated through the sense of taste. As Howes and Lalonde put it, although the English affair with taste "did nothing for British cuisine (that remains as bland as ever)" it did something "for those who thought they had 'taste'; it permitted them to individuate themselves." In this way, the sense of taste in eighteenth-century England functioned very much like the sense of smell did in the late nineteenth-century American South: both putatively premodern and supposedly demoted senses were deemed superior to sight because ruling classes (and races) understood them to be more reliable in fixing identities in rapidly modernizing societies.[15]

Recent work by historians of commodities and food have added much needed detail to this larger framework and, in the process, has extended and refined our understanding of just how indebted national and ethnic identities were to taste in the modern world. We now know, for example, that the Age of Discovery, the systematic settling and exploitation of large parts of Africa, Asia, and the Americas, was also a revolution in taste, especially for the Europeans involved in the extended project. New foods – and tastes – deluged Europe. Potatoes, tomatoes, maize, various peppers, chocolate or cacao, and various fruits all introduced new tastes and were incorporated into prevailing standards and beliefs. Other tastes and commodities migrated in ways that muddied their provenance. Sugar, for example, was of Old World origin, as were coffee and tea. Sugar cane in particular, already known to Europeans, migrated to the New World where it was cultivated on such a scale that it inundated European markets (in the form of molasses and rum as well as sugar) and, as a result, became associated with the taste of the New World.[16]

The introduction of sugar into the European diet on a large scale beginning in the seventeenth century was momentous in many respects, changing what people tasted and the way they tasted. "Until the seventeenth century," explains Sidney W. Mintz, "ordinary folk in Northern Europe secured sweetness in food mostly from honey and from fruit." Although processed cane sugar was being produced in and around the Mediterranean in the eighth century, it was expensive, largely medicinal in its use, and certainly too modest in its supply to be consumed by any but the most affluent. The processing of cane sugar in the New World changed this. English sugar consumption alone increased fourfold between 1640–1700 and then doubled again by the end of the eighteenth century when per capita consumption stood at a staggering thirteen pounds. Remarkably, levels continued to increase in the nineteenth and twentieth centuries, especially in Britain but also in the United States.[17]

Although sugar consumption levels were not the same everywhere – Britain preferred it more than France – Mintz considers sugar "unmistakably modern" for three reasons: it was among the first edible luxuries to become commonplace among the working classes; it was among the first commodities to become considered essential by the people who had not produced it; and sugar, like coffee also, was among "the first substances to become the basis of advertising campaigns to increase consumption." Sugar was also handy for New World plantation owner and European industrial capitalist alike: the former used slaves to produce it and profited handsomely; the latter likely smiled as workers consumed it since sugar was a source of cheap energy, a "proletarian hunger-killer." The introduction of sugar into northern Europe also profoundly affected what people now considered relatively "sweet" and relatively tart.[18]

In North America itself, the Age of (Gustatory) Discovery gave way to the Age of (Gustatory) Exchange as Native Americans, various European groups – notably the English, Dutch, French, and Spanish – and West Africans encountered one another as consumers and producers of particular foods and tastes. Each group had a history of adapting to foods, although some were better positioned than others when it came to exchanging culinary practices and the tastes that accompanied them. Native Americans especially "enjoyed tremendous advantages" in this respect, with their knowledge of the land and climate. Corn was their staple grain and provided two-thirds of Native Americans' calories. It was a food eaten by all, gendered in its preparation – women's work – and it was used in a wide variety of ways, ranging from porridges and stews to drinks. Native Americans did not necessarily agree on what constituted "good taste," of course, not least because they were hardly a uniform group. Region mattered and shaped which foods were consumed and, especially, how they were prepared.[19]

New World flora and fauna, topography, and climate challenged European arrivals and they had to adapt their cuisine and tastes accordingly. This, according to Donna R. Gabaccia, is precisely what they did, and successfully, too. "English and French traditions of mixed agriculture," she argues, "proved quite transplantable to the East Coast of North America, allowing European settlers to continue to eat many of their familiar foods." For their part, West Africans "had already adapted their eating to New World crops" prior to their enslavement and subsequent traffic across the Atlantic. Explains Gabaccia: "By 1700 West Africans regularly ate and cultivated corn, cassava, peppers, sweet potatoes, pineapples, and peanuts from the Americas as well as rice and coconuts from Asia." En route to the New World, the enslaved were often fed food grown in their ultimate destination, the taste of slavery polluting their tongues miles before they ever set foot on land. And once in North America, Africans left their culinary mark on the culture at large, especially in slaveholding areas where the enslaved cooked for whites, altered European diets, and fundamentally introduced new ways of eating food. Not only did they bring expertise in, for example, rice growing methods, they also cooked rice in ways that influenced European tastes and consumption patterns as with, for example, the blend of beans and rice known as hoppin' john.[20]

On the whole, no one cuisine won out in colonial America. Foods, cooking styles, and the tastes that accompanied them were traded to produce a distinctly American creole cuisine. Colonial America was a time and place laden with violent conflict and an aggressive construction of difference by Europeans especially. Foodways, though, were not a major part of this story, at least according to Gabaccia. Culinary creolization solidified an American identity and created an American palate of tastes and patterns of consumption that marked them as distinctive, a product not of one society but, rather, of several. It was a distinctness that fed, literally and symbolically, American notions of national identity during the American Revolution and after. "The only way to become an American, at least as an eater," argues Gabaccia, "was to eat creole – the multi-ethnic cuisine of a particular region."[21]

A different interpretation, one more attuned to subtleties of tension and conflict, is offered by James E. McWilliams and reveals how food was contested and taste reconfigured as part of the process of cultural adaptation and domination in North America. For McWilliams, the first white settlers decried Indian corn as a "heathan graine," one they had encountered before settling North America, courtesy of explorers and the Spanish in the sixteenth century. The English considered corn unfit for people and better suited to animals, which is why, in the initial instance, they used it to feed swine. And yet, by 1650, the English in colonial North America were happily eating cornmeal. Regardless of region, regardless of class, corn was now a staple part of the North American diet. Yet the "exchange," such as it was, proved a trade among unequals and was inscribed by colonial statements on the part of the English about good taste and the need to reconfigure Indian corn so that it became palatable and, in fact, non-Indian.[22]

Such was the case with New Englanders especially who adopted the grain but on their own terms. "Corn would work," notes McWilliams, "as long as it didn't upset the goal of replicating the agricultural ways of the homeland." New Englanders grew corn in a meticulous, precise, agricultural fashion, quite unlike what they perceived as the hasty clearing of brush and scattering of seed employed in the Indian manner. Settlers also diluted the Indianness of corn by incorporating it into a number of English culinary practices. Most obviously, they "anglicized" corn by using it to brew beer. In this way, corn and other Indian foods gradually became incorporated into English ways of eating and tasting.[23]

And once the taste of Indian food had become anglicized, so English food – European food generally – was reconstituted as American during the Revolution. Food, at least for white Americans, was central to the elaboration of American identity and national consciousness during and, especially after, the Revolution. Predictably and unimaginatively – but nonetheless successfully – Americans styled their food in opposition to various European cuisines, most notably the English and French. Framed squarely within the prevailing idiom of republican simplicity and frugality, Americans claimed their cuisine reflected their common values, stressing rusticity, plainness, lacking in pretension, and deeply connected to the land. Americans preferred their "frugal plain repast," not the "high seasoned food" of Europeans and cast their taste in a vernacular of culinary homespun. They liked to eat "pompkin pie," "cranberry sauce," a simple, easy pot pie (frequently contrasted with the more involved and complicated English mince pie), and, of course, that once loathed but now loved staple of Indian pudding and cornmeal. American taste was thoroughly political, from beginning to end.[24]

The sense of taste, in fact, received something of a boost from modernity and continued to inform some of its fundamental categories, nationalism especially. As trade became more extensive and goods, information, and people began to circulate with increasing speed and over greater distances in the nineteenth and twentieth centuries, tastes increasingly migrated too, encountering one another in new ways, sometimes accommodating, sometimes clashing, and often informing migrant and immigrant identities in powerful ways. What little work that has been done on this topic is usually indirect and implicit but, nonetheless, suggestive and revealing. David Sutton, for example, has found how Greek identity – local and familiar at one level but also thoroughly national at another – was maintained among Greek Diaspora communities in the twentieth century through the consumption – gustatory and olfactory – of distinctly Greek foods. Greeks continued to consume national foods partly in an effort to minimize a sense of dislocation and partly to reconstruct their sense of wholeness. "Food," observes Sutton, "is essential to counter tendencies toward fragmentation of experience" and taste and associated smells were central to the reconstitution of Greek identity in an increasingly transglobal world in the late twentieth century. For decades, Greek immigrants who left Greece, no matter their location, bought olive oil to remind them of their homes, used global mail serves to shuttle foods from Greece to their new location and thereby relocated their sense of national identity and their past ("eating the past," Sutton calls it), all of which helped temper the emotional burden and feeling of *xenitia*, or exile in a foreign land. The preservation and elaboration of ethnic and national identity through food, cooking, and the use of particular ingredients might well apply to every group that has migrated throughout history, not just the Greeks, and attention to the historical importance to taste in this context could help us better understand how the senses have informed modern ideas about ethnicity and national identity.[25]

The role of taste in creating and inscribing identities, local and national, was by no means an exclusively Western phenomenon. National tastes and tastes of nationalism played an important role in twentieth-century China, a role made apparent through the history of monosodium glutamate, or MSG. Often understood in the West as a source of burning sensations and headaches following a meal in a Chinese restaurant, the history of this widely used flavor enhancer reveals with wonderful precision the contours of what historian Karl Gerth has described as China's "battle to break free from imperialist control during the decades before the Communist revolution in 1949." China's efforts to produce, market, and consume a domestic version of imported MSG was central to what Gerth terms "nationalistic commodification," in the case of MSG a way to consume and taste modern ideas about nationalism and Chinese identity. China's National Products Movement, established between the end of the last dynasty in 1911 and the re-emergence of a strong state under Chiang Kai-shek in 1927–1928, was designed to invest national identity in products. MSG was one such product.[26]

A good deal of MSG's association with Chinese national identity is attributable to the activities – and cultural representation of – Wu Yunchu, Chinese entrepreneur and scientist. Wu's production and marketing of his MSG as authentically and meaningfully "Chinese" was so successful at weaning China from an earlier, Japanese-manufactured MSG that the Communist Chinese leadership recognized his contribution to modern national identity, formally confirming his title as *minzu zibenzhuyi* or "MSG King" in 1950. Wu and his biographers, all of whom stressed his Chinese origins, managed to braid the taste of MSG with national identity by stressing the deep historical genealogy of Chinese use of the enhancer (while MSG entered U.S. households in the 1950s, a cognate – seaweed – had been used for thousands of years in East Asia generally) and, critically, by making the consumption of Wu's MSG an act of patriotism and an active rejection of the imported, Japanese, increasingly "foreign," and, in Wu's opinion, less tasty, version. Wu was so successful that in the 1930s he began exporting MSG and, in effect, gave the world a carefully constructed "taste" of China.[27]

Taste, cuisine, and food functioned in other ways in China to shape national identity. As Mark S. Swislocki has shown in his study of food culture in Republican Shanghai (1912–1949), Chinese social critics frequently indexed personal diets and food consumption to the health of the nation generally. Responsibility for national health, for workers and elites alike, rested with the housewife who was obliged to feed her family so that the nation might thrive. Here, as in ancient Greece, women seem to have been associated with the sense of taste. In Republican Shanghai, a city with a stunning variety of cuisines arranged along ethnic, class, and regional tastes, food, despite its gustatory variety, was standardized in the service of the modern political state. Food took on overtly political meanings, at least in official conversations. Food fed bodies and strong bodies were necessary for a strong state, so the argument went. In this respect, food was rendered a tasteless political question, a purely biomedical affair linking the Chinese body to the body politic. What should and should not be eaten mattered not in terms of taste but in terms of diet and what was "good" for you and, by extension, the state.[28]

Modernity – in the form of a self elaborated and proclaimed cosmopolitism – was also used by individual cities. Shanghai of the 1920s and 1930s was home to every Chinese regional taste and, as such, fashioned itself as a gustatory microcosm of the national palate which in turn was marked by its diversity. In addition to restaurants catering to international cuisines – American and French, notably – Shanghai offered multiple regional cuisines, at once feeding off of and helping create gustatory associations. The city could satisfy northerners' putative penchant for scallions and garlic, the Hunanese and Sichuanese taste for hot and spicy, and "stinky foods" supposedly adored by the Shaoxing people, among others.[29]

Class identity was part and parcel of the creation of China's national cuisine and what one tasted – and how – was very much contingent on social standing and economic wealth in Shanghai. Wealthier families tended to eat out in restaurants in the 1930s, and thus had the opportunity to expose their palates to a genuinely flourishing international cuisine (it was possible to taste cuisines from a number of countries in Shanghai). Modernity – understood as a discursive rather than analytic category – was, in part, tasted and manifest in the variety of foods and how they were consumed according to class in the city. Working people ate largely at home, relied heavily on rice, and economized wherever possible, buying, for example, white bean or vegetable oil rather than more expensive peanut oil. Material needs shaped what was cooked and how and gave the food a markedly "working class" taste. But choices were made: workers tended to spend a good proportion of their income on wine and cigarettes and considered such tastes distinctive gustatory pleasures. Upper- and middle-class families also exercised gustatory choice and reaffirmed their class identity by buying different kinds of food, often from markets in more Westernized parts of Shanghai and adopting a more Western diet. Cattle beef – as opposed to water buffalo or ox – was prized by such families and could be obtained only in the Western markets. The amount of beef consumed did not serve as a way to delineate taste among classes, but the type of beef consumed did.[30]

Perhaps because food was – and is – physiologically necessary, the sense of taste was an extremely fugitive sense and it can be found functioning not simply as nourishment but as a way to inform class identities in any number of societies outside of China. Urbanization and attendant class formation in nineteenth-century France, for example, generated complicated gustatory stereotypes that helped fracture the lower orders. The Parisian working class – increasingly urbanized, time-disciplined, and used to an urban diet – felt "nothing but contempt" for rural workers who ate at haphazard times, without cutlery, and exhibited a "peasant taste in food." The method and temporal discipline of food consumption was, in both nineteenth- and twentieth-century France, an esthetic governing social class that was almost as important as the actual taste of food and the choice of meal. Taste was also important for elaborating class identities and ethnic affiliations, even in societies that rhetorically claimed to have ended those distinctions. When Russians were required to work with Kazakh laborers in the building of vast railroads under Stalinist rule in the 1920s, ethnic tension was sometimes, literally, a matter of taste. Russians, for example, taunted Kazakhs – largely Muslims – by smearing pig fat on their lips or forcing them to eat pork. Coerced taste was a serious attempt to negate Kazakh identity.[31]

Taste and Truth

If taste, especially in the form of cuisine and food consumption, helped anchor and elaborate national identity and class and ethnic distinctions generally in the modern era in many parts of the world, it also proved a malleable yet quite tenacious sense, a point with which I'd like to conclude. While it is clear that, since the Enlightenment, taste as well as vision inscribed identities at all levels, it was also a very plastic sense, subject to frequent and important redefinitions of what taste meant and how it functioned as an authenticator of truth and generator of reliable knowledge.

A sense of taste – one defined by a community, not by individual or judicial standards – was very much in play following a serious contamination of water in the Canadian town of Walkerton, Ontario, which killed seven people in 2000–2002, as Joy Parr has shown. Water contamination profoundly affected how people both in Walkerton and far removed from the town began to doubt the ability of taste to anchor certainty – in this case, whether or not good water could be verified by the tongue. According to Parr, parts of this story relate to the larger questions of interest to historians of the sensorium. Parr explains: "it is about daily learning of the keynotes of a place – the common smells, the wind, the strength of the 'natural' light – that come to indwell as organizing instruments for cognitive processing, without being spoken. This knowledge that evades the discursive and depends on merged perceptions processed by sight, touch, hearing, and, as I came to recognize as I followed the Walkerton instance, by taste and smell." The "taste" of Walkerton's groundwater had long been a matter of local pride and importance – Walkerton's water was considered to have a distinctive flavor (thus anchoring taste to place) and local residents were deemed to be the best judges not only of the water's esthetic taste but also its goodness, its safety. The corruption of the water source and the resulting deaths remade taste in Walkerton. Residents could not trust their tongues to detect the *E. coli* contamination of their water supply, despite their ardent belief in their power of taste. After the outbreak, only scientific verification of the water's safety by officials external to the town could guarantee its safety. The idea of taste was remade quickly, undermining at once the sovereignty of place, "locally embedded knowledge," and the authority of local tongues. Plainly, modernity had not wholly erased the importance people in Walkerton attached to taste in 2000, but the contamination of the water supply showed that taste was no longer a wholly reliable arbiter. Only scientists from afar could be entrusted to define what was good and bad water; local tongues no longer functioned reliably in that role. In other words, it was not print that diluted the power of taste here; rather, it was what Parr calls "the late modern assessment of risk," who defines risk and how. What is perhaps most revealing in this episode, however, is not simply how the prerogatives of local taste became undermined; rather, it is how very tenacious the sense of taste proved as an arbiter of truth. Although, in a general sense, the modern processing of food and technologies allowing people to freeze and "cook" food within minutes has tended to dilute taste as a mode of knowing, taste in Walkerton was still very much believed to be a reliable detector of knowledge. It took a significant and wrenching event to destabilize taste's authenticating role but the destabilization occurred not in the seventeenth or eighteenth century but, rather, at the dawn of the twenty-first.[32]

5

Touching

Getting in Touch with the Past

Any gesture toward sensory history would do well to recall that the saying "seeing is believing" is a shortened version of the original old English formulation, "seeing is believing, but feeling's the truth." According to Constance Classen, scholars especially should keep the saying in mind because they can be indifferent to the importance of touch as a critical part of historical experience. "Rather than grasping an issue," remarks Classen, "academics shed light on it. Rather than taking a stand, they have a point of view," and rather than touch on or weigh problems, they search for perspective and offer focus. There is no small irony here: the products of scholarship, the very products of the print revolution – books – have not always been wholly visual in nature. Books, form their inception, held a profoundly tactile quality. Books were, and are, held, carried, opened, thumbed, fingered, and stroked, at least in C. S. Lewis's estimation. The act of writing itself has always been a deeply tactile experience (pens and pencils are held, keys on boards are tapped).[1]

The general indifference toward hapticity plays up the idea that touch was variously more carnal, lewd, primitive, emotional, and less intellectual than sight. This assumption has proved so enduring not least because it has such a deep, almost unfathomable genealogy. Plato and Aristotle agreed that touch was radically inferior to sight and the idea that tactility was bereft of intellectual context lasted, according to some interpretations, well into the Middle Ages and beyond. The sense of touch, at least in the way that some writers and intellectuals have perceived it, seems to have changed very little from antiquity to the present.[2]

The dearth of historical work on tactility has not escaped those interested in initiating a sustained historical treatment of the topic. In her insightful brief on the nature of sensory history and its likely development, Joy Parr remarks that she is "most interested in and daunted by the haptic" and recognizes that historians of touch have few signposts to help them. "We might," she reasonably suggests, "expect histories of dance, sport, and architectural design to be rich in example and vocabulary through which to study the haptic. I have not found them so." Indeed, compared to literary, anthropological, and philosophical treatments of hapticity, historical work on touch generally is relatively rare, virtually all of it in European history, and a good deal of it indebted to literary scholars and historians of medicine.[3]

To be fair, I suspect that the historical study of touch has been slighted because of the difficulty in coming to terms with the sense. As Sander Gilman, one of the few historians to have done serious work on touch, remarks, "The study of touch is made difficult because it is at the same time the most complex and the most undifferentiated of the senses. Sight, hearing, smell and taste all have specific, limited sensory organs, all of which have specific limited functions." By contrast, according to Gilman, the skin "is not only an organ of sense but it serves as the canvas upon which we 'see' touch and its cultural associations."[4] This can lead, as with Gilman's own work, to, ironically enough, understanding tactility through sight and importing a visualist idiom to something that was, while obviously seen, also felt. Gilman maintains: "To comprehend the social construction of 'touch' and its relationship to sexuality, we must take into consideration the fact that the representation of touch is always in the realm of another sense, that of sight, whether it is the 'seeing' of the text representing sexuality, or the 'seeing' of touch." Gilman argues for linking tactility and sight and he is correct to do so. But there is some danger in doing so and small conceptual missteps might eclipse the very sense we seek to understand. Writes Gilman: "Since culturally we do not record our icons on our skin but only through the organ of sight we need to link these two senses to write our history of the erotic touch. Thus the status afforded sight and touch, most often considered the highest and the lowest of the senses, is not random." True enough, but the historian of tactility must always be keenly alert to evidence that depicts feeling and tactility, not just how skin was seen, as important part of the story though that is.[5]

Recently, things have been looking up for touch. Scholarly treatments have become more common in recent years, so that while there is an enormous amount of research still left to be done, we now possess at least an adumbration of a social and cultural history of touch and much of it is now being properly historicized. While Sander Gilman was, in 1993, correct to argue that a good deal of "scholarly interest in the recent past in the history of touch has been ... focused on the biology of touch, rather than in its representation," most work now attempts to get to grips with touch by treating it as historically situated.[6]

More than that, a good deal of recent work has shown how touch and skin has "been indulged and catered to in modernity." Tactility and consciousness of skin – how it looks, its color, its feel – has proven essential to the elaboration of modern ideas and processes, from the construction of gender, race, and class to the blueprinting of ideas concerning comfort, pain, and capitalism. "The modern world is supposedly a domain of visibility, constituted by the hegemony of the gaze, governed by panoptic surveillance," writes David Chidester, elaborating: "But modernity is also tactility." Tactility was deeply implicated in modernity and the task for the historian is to show how protocols of touch, meanings of hapticity, and ideas surrounding touch and skin changed over time rather than accepting the easy and largely undocumented claim that the rise of print and the Enlightenment greatly reduced touch's importance.[7]

By the same token, we should not necessarily assume that tactility in early non-Western societies was wholly "premodern." Take, for example, the link between the written word and skin apparent in the early modern Chinese practice of *ling chi*, a punishment known as "death by slicing." The earliest references to the punishment are from 1028 and the practice apparently flourished under the Sung dynasty (960–1279) sponsored by scholar-gentry rulers who replaced the old aristocracy. The punishment was used especially for bandits and those found guilty of treason and religiously inspired murders. According to one source, the offender's skin was sliced a thousand times, with every ten cuts announced to gathered crowds. In effect, the punishment of the state was written onto the skin of the body. After 1,000 cuts, the body was dissected into 3,600 pieces, the approximate number of characters a Chinese person needed to know to read and write. Literacy was deeply connected to skin, sight to tactility, the punishment of the skin perhaps an effort to "civilize" errant bandits in the ways of the scholar-gentry, all of which muddies tidy connections between writing, seeing, touching, and modernity.[8]

The Pre-Enlightened Touch

There was not an undifferentiated sense of touch in that huge swathe of time referred to as "premodernity," the period stretching from antiquity to the Enlightenment, at least in the West. Touch during antiquity and the medieval period in the West was implicated in virtually every aspect of life, giving shape to social, political, and cultural relations, playing a major role in transcending earthly and spiritual worlds, and informing the operation and workings of any number of disciplines.

Touch was a critical, authenticating sense in some ancient and early modern legal systems, for example. Bernard Hibbitts has found that "unilateral gentle touching can communicate the assertion of legal authority over another person or thing," such as with the early Roman procedure in which masters claimed ownership of slaves by touching them with a ceremonial rod or as with dying men touching the hand of their preferred heir in ancient Mesopotamian law. Mesopotamians also announced legal claims and accusations by hitting or slapping foreheads, a practice that was continued in early medieval Europe where knighthood could be conferred on a squire through a smack on the face or neck, precursor to the gentler dubbing with the sword. Kissing played an important role in marking legal and social bonds, especially in some European feudal societies and, in early medieval German law, a lord could reclaim a serf by holding his coat-tail. Commercial deals were sealed in feudal France and Germany through the striking of palms and medieval vassals commonly placed their hands within their lord's to indicated submission to his feudal prerogative.[9]

So too with medicine. Galenic medicine stressed the importance, even indispensability, of touch in reading pulse and temperature and in palpitating the body. Humoral medicine was very much framed within tactile coordinates and often pointedly gendered. Men's skin – and, by extension, the feel of their touch – was believed to be dry and hot in nature, women were pejoratively cold and moist, a product of "undercooked" semen. Heat – felt through the skin – was a sign of strength while cold reflected weakness. Non-Western medicine also relied heavily on touch, albeit with subtle differences from early Western practices. Siddha medicine, one of India's traditional medical systems elaborated between the tenth and fifteenth centuries, was heavily indebted to touch. In contrast to Western biomedicine's emphasis on the single diastolic-systolic touch, the Siddha physician distinguished between six pulses and also used his fingertips to sense differential pressures. Although British medical systems were introduced in colonial

India, Siddha emphasis on tactility as an authenticating sense remained important and does so to this day.[10]

Arguably, though, nowhere was tactility more important than in elaborating religious beliefs. Touching for early Christians, for example, was linked to both pain and pleasure, less as a binary and more as a whole, a tactile continuum in which pain and pleasure were joined. Early Christians kissed one another in holy salute (although the rule later changed so that men kissed only men and women only women to avoid sexual suggestion) and the tactile dimensions of religion lasted into the medieval period. In Alain de Lille's *Anticlaudianus* of 1183, touch is understood as the force "the Mother of the Gods gave to Nature and with it the Knot of Love was tied tighter and bound their vows." Little wonder that early medieval pilgrims sought to validate faith by touching statues and relics. Tactility was, in short, inextricable to the articulation and fulfillment of Christian faith.[11]

Touch as marker of hierarchy was deeply connected to early Christian images of God's touch. A number of eleventh-century European bibles, for example, depict God as sculptor, fashioning Adam with his hands, or show him simply touching Adam's shoulder. Yet Adam never touches God since man's touch in this context was not only irrelevant but likely smacked of misguided notions of equality. Similar images populate a number of fourteenth-century European cathedral carvings and in each instance the notion that touch through hands can animate or create is clear.[12]

The ascetic tradition in Christianity was also very skin-sensitive. Sin could caress flesh, pricking it to lust; it could also be countered through the imposition of bodily pain. The Flagellant Movement in twelfth- and thirteenth-century Europe introduced this idea into popular culture. Flagellants traveled from town to town scourging themselves, reminding themselves – and their viewers – of Christ's sacrifice and death. The idea reached its clearest articulation with Saint Ignatius Loyola who counseled that spiritual attentiveness was facilitated not simply through the exaggerated infliction of pain through flagellation but through daily, hourly tactile reminders, in part achieved by "wearing hairshirts or cords or iron chains."[13]

In his study of mystical language and the senses in the late Middle Ages, Gordon Rudy finds that a key feature associated with modernity – a sensory construction of self – was achieved through the deployment of putatively premodern senses, especially taste and touch. Theologically, the relationship between a transcendent god, something beyond body, and the senses was discussed in detail by Origen of Alexandria

(c. 185–252) who did much to establish the doctrine of the spiritual senses. Spiritual senses, argued Origen, belonged to the inner life and allowed people to come to know spirituality, especially God. Origen's doctrine operated at the intersection of religious and bodily beliefs about the nature of God and was elaborated and refined by a number of writers in the twelfth, thirteenth, and fourteenth centuries, notably the twelfth-century Cistercian monk Bernard of Clairvaux (1090–1153), Hadewijch of Brabant (a Dutch holy woman, fl. 1230–1250), Bonaventure, the Franciscan theologian (1221–1274), and the Flemish theologian, Jan van Ruusbroec (1293–1381). Although these writers revised Origen and other theologians, and while "they tended to blur the distinctions between body and soul or spirit ... and between the self and God", they nonetheless understood the self to be an operational category in a spiritual sense that could understand God through taste and touch.[14]

The growing interest in the supposedly "lower" senses of taste and touch and their spiritual significance in the late Middle Ages is quite important, not least because, according to Rudy at least, theologians prior to the twelfth century generally remained very suspicious of injecting these lower senses into religious discussions, much preferring to frame spiritual understanding exclusively within the intellectual senses of sight and hearing. In this respect, the more chronologically "premodern" the theologian, the more ardent his or her commitment to the higher senses of sight and sound. In the Middle Ages, theologians increasingly turned to the putatively lower, premodern senses of taste and touch especially to come to terms with profoundly theological matters, some of which centered on the idea of one's self and its relation to God. These later theologians qualified Origen's exclusively spiritual understanding of the senses to focus on the bodily senses and the human Jesus – his pain, hunger, suffering – in short, his sensory, corporeal meaning which, at the time, was being elaborated in monastic European culture especially. From here, the idea of an intimate, sensory relationship with God gained currency.[15]

Bernard of Clairvaux frequently discussed union with God employing ideas of taste and touch and was careful to show how the senses intertwined. He maintained, for example, according to Rudy, that those "who acquire faith by hearing can 'touch' God in Christ and 'taste' wisdom and contemplation." Rudy comments that although some medieval theologians believed that God could not be seen in his unapproachable brightness, Bernard argued: "faith reaches the unreachable, catches the unknown, grasps what cannot be measured, takes hold of the uttermost, and in a way encompasses even eternity itself in its broad breast." Fascinatingly, Rudy interprets this to mean: "Bernard inverts the traditional hierarchy: he places sight first and *lowest*, taste and touch last and *highest*" in an effort to "articulate the immediacy and mutuality of union with God." Here, touch especially functioned as faith: to truly touch the hem of Jesus' cloak demanded faith and divine wisdom, reciprocity between God and individual. Wisdom, in turn, was tasted and considered superior to matters that were only "seen." Wrote Bernard: "by tasting discover and judge how sweet the Lord is." Hadewijch made similar and, in some respects, even more pointed claims about the centrality of taste and touch to faith and the individual's relationship with God while for others, such as the early thirteenth-century Parisian theologian William of Auxerre, God's understanding of charity was distinctly tactile. On the whole, many medieval theologians viewed spiritual senses as other-worldly and earthly, serving to consummate man's knowledge of God, and touch was deeply relevant to the form and meaning of that knowledge.[16]

Haptic Modernity

Gender and Violence

As with hearing and smelling, as well as sight, touching was inextricable to the elaboration of a post-Renaissance and post-Enlightenment Western world. Ideas concerning hapticity proved incredibly important for all sorts of developments during and long after the invention of print and the dissemination of print culture and reading habits.

This is not to suggest that the Renaissance itself generally had no effect on ideas concerning tactility. What had been a fairly stable tactile image in early Christian iconography became muddied with secularization. Ideas of touch became increasingly visual during the Renaissance, giving rise to what Sander Gilman calls the "fantasy of 'seeing' the sense of touch," already commonplace in the seventeenth century. An important development between the Middle Ages and the Renaissance concerning the "social implications of the association between sexuality and touch" helps account for this. For Gillman, the incursion of sight into tactility resided in "the great syphilis epidemic of the late fifteenth and early sixteenth centuries" which rendered "the sexualized touch also the sign of death." Touch was now linked to concerns over pollution in the form of disease and sexuality and, increasingly, depicted visually in artwork.[17]

Tactility's association with disease and sex denigrated the sense, and the Enlightenment further discounted touch, especially when it came to establishing truth and ferreting out meaning. By the time intellectuals such as Johann Wolfgang von Goethe began to think seriously about the nature of touch, its sexual components, its duality as toucher and touched, and its esthetic qualities in the 1790s, "the construction of touch as a social and intellectual category as the lowest of the senses had a long intellectual history." Also in the eighteenth century, Immanuel Kant deliberated on the sense of touch and helped seal its fate as the lowest sense. For Kant, touch was quite empirical because it was a physical sense but its very directness made it the custodian and courier of unreflected and unexamined knowledge. Sight, conversely, Kant considered thoroughly detached, distanced, and inherently reflective. Thus did touch by the end of the eighteenth century become the sense associated "with the irrational, with the direct, unreflected, physically proximate comprehension of the world."[18]

Yet Kant and other intellectuals cleaved to an understanding of the world that failed to take account of its lived sensory complexity. For example, the argument that the Enlightenment's association with seeing owed much to an increasingly visual emphasis in medicine is misleading, at least if we are to believe recent work by cultural historians of medicine generally and of early modern midwifery in particular. The binary model of sight as rational and modern and touch as irrational and premodern lacks the nuance and flexibility to account for a number of medical practices becoming popular in eighteenth-century England. Increasingly, male midwives and male surgeons reconstituted touch – at least *their* touch – as rational and scientific as long as their male hands were doing the touching. Edmund Chapman, an influential London surgeon who wrote an *Essay on the Improvement of Midwifery* in 1733 attempted to undermine the tactile authority of female midwives by casting their touch as clumsy and emotional. By contrast, maintained Chapman, the touch of the man of medicine was scientifically probing, decorously rational, and able to generate important medical knowledge. In this respect, male physicians and surgeons and male midwives reconstituted touch as rational and professional, a source of knowledge and truth, by gendering it, by making their touch intellectual work and the touch of the female midwife overly aggressive, unreliable, likely to do more harm than good to newborns and laboring mothers, and typical of rough, unrefined manual labor. The effect was twofold. First, tactility became an important part of medical practice and midwifery, even at the height of Enlightenment thinking about retinal preeminence, and, second, it served to help undermine women's position as caregivers, members of the medical community, and midwives, while promoting men in those roles, including, obviously, obstetrics. Women resisted such trends and some men objected too on the grounds that male midwives were really touching for sexual, not professional, reasons. But the reconstitution of the medical touch as scientific, legitimate, and as a way for male physicians especially to establish protocols regarding the right to touch bodies in a professional capacity emerged even as vision become increasingly important to framing modernity.[19]

While patriarchy was often reinforced through touch, so too were power distinctions among women. As Laura Gowing argues, "Women's authority in neighborhood and household made itself felt, very often through touch. Women pushed and nudged each other, shared beds, touched each other's breasts, or felt bellies. Physical intimacies and confrontations made solid the distinctions of status and age that divided women." Touch policed behavior and the body and functioned in the early modern West not unlike sight supposedly did in the modern era.[20]

All of this amounted to what Gowing calls a "politics of touch." Between men, the distance of "span" – nine inches – was, in polite circles, considered gentlemanly and appropriate, a mark of civility. Men of any rank, however, saw the female body as always open to touch and, therefore, possession. Men could and did push women, rub against, hit, and sexually assault them in private and public. The marital status and age of the woman mattered, though, and married women were not touched as much in inappropriate ways as were single, younger women by men. But older, married women and women in positions of power also used touch to in part prop up patriarchy and also to reaffirm their own status. Servant girls found their bodies violated, pushed, abused sexually, by masters and mistresses; poor, young, pregnant women had their bodies felt, prodded, and invaded by the hands of female midwives who used tactility not just to read and understand the pregnant woman's condition but also to assert their authority and power as older women.[21]

Men, too, abused one another and, in the process, revealed assumptions about skin, masculinity, and class. In nineteenth-century America, especially in southern and western states, for example, elite British and northern travelers commented extensively on the viciousness of physical violence among poor whites. For poor white men, manliness and social status were measured very much in haptic terms – how much punishment the skin could take, how much violence it could dish out. In this world, cast as thoroughly uncivilized by American and British elites, skin sometimes trumped eyes. Gouging was extremely common – finger nails were sharpened especially to facilitate a quick popping of an opponent's eye in a fight. Horrified bourgeois spectators from American urban regions, especially the modernizing northeast, shuddered at the sight of hands and fingers denigrating vision in a very real sense. With the American Civil War, such frontier violence changed to a more visual, less tactile form of violence, one facilitated by the rapid and widespread dissemination of handguns and rifles. Killing and violence was now done more often at a distance, courtesy of a steady eye, not a toughened or calloused hand or filed nail. In this instance, vision did indeed come to displace and dilute touch. Even when physical violence was condoned by elites and, as with boxing, sponsored by them, bare knuckles – skin against skin – were replaced with gloves (the 1867 Queensberry Rules called for the wearing of gloves and the 1839 London Prize Ring Rules outlawed gouging). That much said, bare-knuckle fighting was never truly erased by bourgeois sensibilities. In fact, the sight of extreme forms of violence – defined especially by the fierce disregard for skin – can still be seen in the popularity of Ultimate Fighting Championships in the United States and bare-knuckle, underground brawls in Britain which, though difficult to measure, have remained more common and popular than is generally recognized.[22]

In Touch with Politics and Political Economy

Although there was a good deal of continuity in the history of touch and meanings of tactility between the premodern and modern periods, modernity and especially what Norbert Elias called the "civilizing process" nevertheless wrought some important changes on how touch was understood. The broad process of instilling restraint, of disciplining the self, which Elias described as the essential component of the emergence of modernity, helped interiorize aspects of touch, tended to relegate ideas of physical touch to the affective realm, and internalize emotion. Tactile table manners, for example, were critically important for the elaboration of custom and social relations in the Middle Ages. Feeding with hands reaffirmed communal social relations and diluted nascent notions of individualism. The Renaissance and the Enlightenment altered the kinds of touch central to social control and authority and stressed the importance of keeping one's hands to oneself. The man of court, for Elias, became controlled, a master of his gestures, his touches framed and choreographed precisely, his interior world impenetrable to the outside viewer. As Elizabeth D. Harvey thoughtfully suggests, "one of touch's discursive transpositions mimics this civilizing trend: in the same way that physical impulses curbed and directed inward, so does tactility become, in addition to the more obvious physiological responses, 'feeling' – the emotional desires and urges that are presented in explicitly physical terms in the early modern iconography of touch."[23]

In other words, touch became extremely orchestrated, directed, disciplined, and emotionally meaningful. At the same time, in eighteenth-century Europe at least, a growing consensus emerged that inner values and character were "written upon the skin." Skin was not simply an organ of sensation it was also a canvass. This function of the skin was critical for helping shape perceptions of class, worth, and character. Eighteenth-century European physiognomists, such as Johann Caspar Lavater, for example, maintained that crude individuals manifested their baseness in the texture of their skin, which was invariably coarse.[24]

The disciplined touch, the revelatory nature of the skin, and the social message conveyed in how one touched and what one touched coalesced in eighteenth- and nineteenth-century ideas about comfort. Eighteenth-century notions of "comfort" in Anglo-America, while certainly indexed to the sense of sight (mirrors, lamps, candles, offered visual comfort), hearing (elites preferred quiet rooms), and taste, were principally associated with the sense of touch. Modern notions of comfort were understood in terms of room temperature – not too hot or too cold – and their effect on the skin, in terms of how comfortable clothing felt, and how the body generally was treated by oneself and others. This idea – that comfort was physical, mediated through the body and touch – was, according to John Crowley's fascinating work, "an innovation of Anglo-American culture," one tied intimately to sensory ideas concerning the body and one that evolved slap-bang in the middle of the American Enlightenment. "Comfort," with all of its sensory underpinnings, was thoroughly implicated in modernity.[25]

The eighteenth-century Anglo-American concern with physical comfort marked a significant shift from earlier definitions of the term. For centuries before the eighteenth century, "comfort" referred to emotional, moral, and spiritual well-being under trying circumstances. "Discomfort" involved sorrow and melancholy but had little connection to physical difficulty. Changes in political economy, reconstituted ideas concerning the differences between luxury and necessity, and the burgeoning trans-Atlantic consumer revolution of the 1700s combined to shift the meaning of comfort from the moral and spiritual to the physical realm. Even the emerging humanitarian sensibility at the end of the eighteenth century was articulated in such terms and the idea that the poor, the enslaved, and the weak should not suffer physical discomfort, that it was the responsibility of the propertied to ensure their basic comfort, that there was, fundamentally, a right to comfort, became an important component of nineteenth-century social reform.[26]

The social expression of this shift can be read in the way people dressed and in the sort of items they bought and used. Although the consumer revolution did reflect a concern with material objects as expressions of taste, of gentility especially, and less with comfort, over the course of the eighteenth century a desire for comfort increasingly shaped consumer choice in what they bought. Comfort, in fact, occupied the middle ground between luxury and necessity and eased the tension between the two. Furniture increasingly catered to ease; clothing was designed to feel good as well as establish status; shoe- and saddle-makers stressed fit; goods generally were intended to help gratify the senses, especially taste and touch. A nation's worth was measured in part by its ability to cater to its peoples' gustatory and tactile comfort. Daniel Defoe boasted that England's "manufacturing people ... eat and drink well, cloath warm, and lodge soft" and generally fared better than the European working poor. Leather shoes slowly replaced bare feet and wooden clogs, cotton clothing came increasingly to caress the skin, and even umbrellas were divested of their French, highly feminine associations and adopted by the British to protect their skin less from the sun and more from soaking, skin-tingling, shiver-inducing rains.[27]

If skin functioned as a political economy with regard to comfort, its more explicit political meaning can be found in the history of political touch generally, handshaking specifically. As Elizabeth D. Harvey argues, we must take seriously the history of the hand especially: "While the identifying feature of tactility in the early modern period is precisely its resistance to being identified with a single organ, the hand nevertheless appears with some regularity as a signifier of touch." The political implications of "pressing the flesh" and handshaking is evidently an essential part of the modern political touchscape; it was also of some consequence in the past. England's Charles II, for example, reputedly used his royal touch on tens of thousands of people in an effort to generate popular support in the seventeenth century (Keith Thomas reports that he touched 90,798 people in nineteen years, 1660–1664, and 1667–1782). But Charles II was exceptional only in the number he touched, not in the use of the hand. For years the King's touch was believed to cure scrofula – lymphatic inflammation around the neck. Edward the Confessor introduced the practice, which reached frenzied levels under Charles II (his Register of Healing has 8,577 entries between May 1682 and April 1683), and declined only after the 1688 Revolution because of its Catholic associations. Queen Anne was, apparently, the last English sovereign to claim and use the power of touch to heal.[28]

The curative touch could still be had, however. Some people ventured abroad to be touched by the exiled Stuarts and there remained a "brisk traffic in the touch pieces given to the sufferer at the royal ceremony, and subsequently worn around the neck as a souvenir or a protective amulet." In terms of public perception, the power was not particularly religious; rather, people considered the monarch's healing power innate, mystical, and related to his royal authority. And kings used it as such. In Keith Thomas's estimation, "Charles II began touching while still in exile and lost no time in exploiting the political possibilities of the healing power after the Restoration. Only a few days after landing in England he touched 600 persons in one sitting."[29]

Such tactile authority and political use of the handshake was not confined to monarchy. Touch in the form of handshaking was already quite a political matter in seventeenth-century colonial America. Quakers, for example, seem to have preferred the handshake as a form of gesture rather than doffing hats and bowing and similar "dirty customs" that they regard as communicating an assumed social relationship they regarded as untrue. Handshaking, by contrast, had something of a democratic ring to it, a rough equality more associated with "true honor."[30] Religion seems to have played a key role in such political formulations. "Tactility," argues David Chidester, "is the fundamental bond of religion." *Religion* has its root in *religare*, meaning "to bind," and that idea of tactility, of connections, covenants, and contracts informed religious faith and its history in America. Seventeenth-century Puritans claimed God's touch – specifically his hand – in divining their history, leading them, by hand, across the sea, and undertaking in America the "great work in hand." For Chidester, "This tactile imagery culminated in the central symbol of covenant," the bond between God and his people, a bond at once pleasurable, painful, and thoroughly haptic. God's hand had helped the Puritans establish "elbow room" on the continent, violently flailing and moving Native Americans even as that very action bonded God and his elect in tactile, covenanted union.[31] Plainly, the idea of faith and the senses was not the sole prerogative of Catholicism.

Given handshaking's deep, textured, even pedigreed history, keen readers of modern political processes were quick to import tactility. The handshake became favored among nineteenth-century politicians anxious to authenticate their common man credentials under burgeoning modern democracies. At the crux of the democratic process in the nineteenth century and the attendant expansion of the franchise, the evolution of political machines, the framing and manipulation of political image, stood the need to persuade people of the desirability that a particular man was suited to public office. Images of touch and feel and skin – all heavily masculine – were central to such appeals and that so many of them were framed visually did little to dilute the political importance of the idea of touch and skin.[32]

No less a figure than Abraham Lincoln used touch to authenticate his common-man credentials, especially as president when he routinely engaged in vigorous handshaking bouts. He shook hands with hundreds of people following his inauguration, not least because voters wanted to touch his skin, to feel what they perceived as his rough, frontier, hardened, hands – hands that captured, in many minds, the ideal behind free wage labor, securing the fruits of labor with one's hands, and the rough and ready frontier democracy that northerners especially liked to use to counterpoint the freedom of their society with the hands-off approach to manual labor of southern slaveholders. Lincoln also shook hands with thousands of Union soldiers during the Civil War, his presidential touch serving to inspire and remind those fighting a war increasingly against slavery of the authenticity of his politics and the nobility of their cause.[33]

Other instances of the politics – and poetics – of touch in modern political systems are sometimes difficult to discern, not least because the eye can lead even the careful historian into thinking that what was, for example, worn was of more visual than haptic importance. In fact, clothing was not simply and singularly visual; it was also tactile by definition, suggesting something important about the wearer's skin and, ergo, about his or her worth and social standing. This association was hardly unique to the modern West. Sumptuary law in eleventh-century China points to a connection between touch, skin, clothing, and class. Only the nobility were permitted to wear black sables and ermine, extremely soft furs that caressed the skin almost imperceptibly; commoners had to make do with less refined sheep, sable, and mole skins. A very similar set of sumptuary laws regulated fur-wearing in late medieval England.[34]

Historians sometimes fail to appreciate the political significance of clothing because they understand it as simply a visual representation and "read" how, for example, American "homespun" or tailored suits functioned as political and social statements in the eyes of contemporaries. While such an emphasis has produced some gloriously thoughtful work, it has, at the same time, helped deaden analytic sensitivity to hapticity. Clothes can, and should, be read inside out as well as from outside in so that the quality and feel of the clothing on the inside, how it was understood to either caress or rub the skin of the wearer by spectators, is appreciated thoroughly.[35]

For example, when George Washington wrote to a London merchant in 1765 that Americans would have to dress in homespun and sacrifice fine-looking – and feeling – clothes if they were to be understood as virtuous, simple, and critics of luxury, he was making a claim about clothes' tactile importance, not simply as visual statements of political sensibility. Homespun was rough, fitting for a self-described toughened, virtuous, and masculine republican skin and just looking could tell you a great deal about interior worth and feeling. This tactile aspect of clothing might explain why Washington wore "the plain buff and blue uniform of a colonel in the Virginia militia" to the second session of the Continental Congress in May 1775. The creation of a "sensory model" for the American Revolution included using clothes to suggest how a republican man's skin felt, how his virtue was tough, even leathery, and immune to the tactile allure of silk and other frivolous, fancy finery. In this respect, Thomas Paine's revolutionary pamphlet was indeed *Common Sense* – that of the ordinary, common, republican.[36]

The politics of clothing and how certain materials felt was apparent in other emerging democratic systems. In nineteenth-century Britain, "fustian," a thick, coarse, rough cloth of twilled cotton with a short nap, was the cloth of choice for those appealing to the English working classes. Following his release from prison in 1841, the Chartist leader, Fergus O'Connor, had a suit made entirely of fustian for the express purpose of signaling comity with his followers. He shared, he told them, their hapticity, reflected in their "fustian jackets" and the "blistered hands" that accompanied a working-class existence. The haptic basis of class consciousness – and its political implications – was not lost on Friedrich Engels who three years later in *The Condition of the Working Class in England* highlighted the role of fustian jackets in promoting class identification.[37]

A Touch of Class

The political use of touch under democratic systems in the nineteenth century barely disguised how elites used tactility to also bolster and elaborate key class distinctions. Elites – fading nineteenth century aristocrats especially – frequently described the emerging bourgeoisie as "coarse" while the middle class in turn perceived the lower orders as "rough." Eighteenth- and nineteenth-century European class distinctions, then, were not just a matter of "taste," they were also a matter of touch. Many urban nineteenth-century elites understood the working classes, who often lived too close for physical comfort, as couriers of coarse manners and disease. The presence of the "great unwashed" rendered the nineteenth-century English bourgeoisie a nervous bunch that managed to avoid touching the masses but maintained a watchful eye on their activities by viewing them from above through windows and balconies. The middle class could look and not be touched.[38]

In some ways, touch anchored the hierarchy of the senses and the social divisions echoing it. According to Alain Corbin, elites perceived those groups in eighteenth- and nineteenth-century France who labored with hands, those who were "in constant contact with the inertia of matter" to be "accustomed to exhausting toil," and "spontaneously capable of feeling with their flesh an animal pleasure produced by contact." Conversely, elites and the emerging bourgeoisie, "thanks to their education in and habit of social commerce, and their freedom from manual labour, were able to enjoy the beauty of an object, demonstrate delicacy, subdue the instinct of the affective senses, and allow the brain to establish a temporal gap between desire and its gratification." In a way, "what was decisive was the degree of delicacy of the hand," argues Corbin – the ability to resist direct contact, to pause and keep a distance versus the submission to tactile impulse, the grasp, the clumsy lunge, the heavy-handedness of handling. French elites and the bourgeoisie commonly proclaimed "the insensitivity of touch of the peasantry; the skin of the tiller of the soil was hardened by labour, when, that is, it was not covered with 'as it were a sort of scale'." Corbin further explains: "The coarseness of this creature enslaved to the soil was in keeping with the portrayal of the whole social scene, though this is not to say that I wish systematically to deny the reality of the individual features which composed it." The tendency toward touching was considered by French elites typically plebeian, "a sign of their closeness to the animal; men and women fought and came together brutally." Aristocrats and the bourgeoisie, by contrast, thought seduction demanded distance, "a visual caress" in Corbin's elegant formulation, a trail of scent or a whisper of perfume, not the ham-fisted grab of a fleshy leg by mucky, calloused hands.[39]

Gender intruded, as it often did, and it is worthwhile recalling how, even briefly. The idea of "ladies' work," for example, was deeply tactile. Handiwork and sewing, so poplar among middle-class women in nineteenth-century Anglo-America, was an alternative to the "dominant masculine visualized aesthetic," which promoted a "tactually oriented aesthetic based on traditional women's work." Women's handiwork was understood as the work of the delicate hand, not of the more masculine eye. Handicrafts – lace, sewing, beadwork, scissorwork – were produced by the hand and were meant to be touched. Yet women managed to imbue their work with such skill and intelligence that they not only safely created their own space for artistic freedom but also made hapticity something other than a lower sense.[40]

Beyond the Color of Race

Race-based slavery – and eighteenth- and nineteenth-century imperial efforts to subjugate natives generally – relied heavily on an evolving association between touch, skin, "color," and disease. Touch, in short, and not just vision or color was central to the very construction of the idea of "race" in the modern world and critical to the ways "race" was used to exploit labor and establish hierarchy.[41]

The daily operations of New World slave societies gave vivid and painful voice to such ideas. In the eighteenth- and nineteenth-century American slave South, for example, slaveholders maintained that blackness was not simply a color but also a tactile condition. Black skin, they argued, was at once thicker and tougher than white skin and, ergo, much better suited to hard manual labor. Technological developments helped redefine and reconfigure some of these tactile stereotypes. The invention of the cotton gin in the 1790s and the subsequent flourishing of cotton as the principle southern staple seems to have led planters to talk more frequently not just about the thickness of black skin but about its dexterous quality. Black hands, they suggested, were tough and leathery but sufficiently flexible to pick cotton. White assumptions about the thickness of black skin also help to make better – if wholly unpalatable – sense of the severity of physical punishment meted out to slaves in the South. Slaves were whipped, often brutally, not least because slaveholders believed that their thicker skin had to be stung and slashed with particular ferocity in order to drive "lessons" home.

In the slaveholders' estimation, tough skin demanded especially harsh punishment to ensure the point be properly understood – and felt.[42]

And lest we doubt the modernity of the haptic construction of race, consider how the association between race, sexuality, and the polluted touch resurfaced with wretched poignancy in the 1980s within the iconography of AIDS. As Sander Gilman argues, AIDS – its cause and communication – was thoroughly implicated in racial stereotypes about black pollution and sexuality. "We have not," concludes Gilman, "come very far from the Renaissance in associating the sense of touch and the image of blackness with the sense of disease."[43]

Colonial and imperial projects could also involve ideas about hapticity. As Scott Manning Stevens has shown, European encounters with Native North American Indians were understood very much in tactile terms. Such instances of "first contact," even if that "contact" was initially visual – Indian bodies were seen from afar at first "sighting" – acquired a haptic quality, in part because the notion of "nakedness" and "naked savage" had such currency in seventeenth- and eighteenth-century promotional and encounter literature. Nakedness worked as allure (skin inviting touch) and repulse (difference and fear of contagion) and, from a broadly construed European perspective, the native body functioned as both "sign and signifier of its own materiality." Critically, the way Europeans understood such encounters (rather than "discoveries") helped shape one of the critical – and modern – developments in European history by challenging the idea of "self" and the category of the individual person. Humanism and the Reformation had helped articulate the idea of selfhood and human agency, and the encounter and finding of "an alien Other laid new demands" on that process. In other words, as Stevens poses the problem and as contemporary Europeans understood it, "did different bodies imply different selves?"[44]

Encountering North American Indians as bodies profiled the importance of skin and touch to the very making of European ideas concerning selfhood. Indians occupied a position that required tactile scrutiny on the part of Europeans. They were not as clearly different as West Africans whose "skin color marked them as other" and inferior. But Native Americans did look different too and, in fact, were perceived initially, at least by Columbus, as physically attractive, with fine bodies. The way that colonizers eventually came to consider Native Americans as "others" was due less to European perceptions of their skin color and more to stereotypes concerning their skin and nakedness. Without apparent decency, went European reasoning, Indians showed their flesh and could do so because their skin was immune to the vicissitudes of the environment and indifferent to temperature. And should Europeans transgress and become intimate with such bodies, their sin, as they understood it, was disease, the pox notably. Efforts on the part of some Native Americans to deploy touch in other ways did little to dilute these tactile stereotypes and beliefs on the part of Europeans. Although Indians in early South Carolina touched the shoulders of newcomers to indicate welcome and assure their safety and while some in the gulf region brushed and caressed the first French explorers, presumably out of interest and to affirm that what they saw was real, such haptic interludes were sidebars to the larger story of the tactile construction of Indian otherness and efforts to preserve and elaborate the European sense of self.[45]

Contested interpretations about skin and its meaning occurred during the course of other imperial encounters, especially in the context of trying to "educate" the "natives." C. E. Tyndale-Biscoe, principal of a British school for Kashmiri Pandit boys, detailed in his history of the school, 1880–1930, how British "educators" and "native" children entertained radically different and competing definitions of how skin should look, feel, and smell. What Tyndale-Biscoe and the British understood as filthy skin, marked by itches, very long dirty fingernails, and unwashed hands and faces, the Kashmiri Pandit students saw as perfectly normal and signs of status within their own culture. For the students, the British themselves were untouchable. An exasperated Tyndale-Biscoe put it this way: "It was no use telling them that they were filthy, for they believed they were clean." The key to the colonial project, then, was radical reeducation: "before they could become clean they had to learn they were dirty." They also had to learn that they were effeminate: their dress, preference for clogs, nose-rings, an aversion to blood, and reluctance to touch leather demanded reeducation along masculine, colonial lines. They were thus taught the "manly" art of boxing and the body-disciplining game of cricket. Of course, the students and colonial subjects generally were supposed to contain their manly aspirations so that they never claimed, let alone grasped, true independence.[46]

Intimate Touches?

Injunctions against not touching were as important as touching itself in the nineteenth and twentieth centuries. Between the 1890s and the 1940s, American children, for example, were kept very much at arms length by their parents, at least judging but the immensely popular counsel in L. E. Holt's *The Care and Feeding of Children*, first published in 1894. Touching babies under six months, rocking them, playing with them Holt deemed not only useless but potentially injurious. Holt was not alone, not least because there was a general belief in the medical community that touching babies over stimulated them and that kissing them helped spread disease (tuberculosis and diphtheria especially). Touching should be limited to bathing and dressing, a quick peck on the forehead at night-time, and a cordial handshake in the morning lest parents set up their children for a lifetime of nervous disorders and general social ineptitude as adults. An overly indulged skin was socially and personally dangerous.[47]

Here, haptic protocols concerning children changed very quickly, highlighting just how rapidly sensory stereotypes can evolve and re-configure. Holt's injunctions against touch were simply part and parcel of a larger Victorian movement against tactility. Not that everyone in Victorian America and England stopped touching. In fact, as Peter Gay has shown, middle-class Victorians were more given to haptic pleasures than popular stereotypes suggest. Not only were the bourgeoisie interested in sex and touch – at least if we are to regard American writer Mabel Loomis Todd as even vaguely typical – but the Victorian middle class seemed to revel in the sensual quality of touch (witness the profusion of carpets in the period) without sexualizing tactility. Also, corporal punishment was the norm at home and school. That much said, there were injunctions against touch – as well as directions on how to touch – at the century's end and they were focused on children. Breast-feeding was in decline at the end of the nineteenth century and admonitions against masturbation were increasingly shrill. In some respects, the period witnessed what Anthony Synnott has referred to as children's disembodiment from their own and parents' bodies. And yet, within just a few decades, Western Europe and American child-rearing practices had, at least after the Second World War, reestablished the centrality of tactile communication in child-rearing. Breastfeeding regained popularity and parents were urged to cuddle, kiss, and show affection to their children. Thus even within one relatively short historical moment – from the 1890s to the 1960s – there were multiple histories of touching – injunctions against, urgings for – and different constituencies (children, adults) were subject to different haptic protocols and, thus, experienced different haptic histories.[48]

Multiple histories of touch are also apparent in even smaller slices of time. Touch was a fundamental part of the meaning, content, and elaboration of the world's first modern war. The German military aimed to make men and soldiers out of boys by subjecting their skin to radical treatments to harden the body and spirit. German military academies beat cadets' bodies, pulled their baby teeth, and generally aimed to masculinize their recruits by creating an armor or "thick skin" which at once made them physically hardened soldiers but also emotionally distant from their affective home life.[49]

But that dreadful war softened those same bodies. The atrocious conditions of the front, the mud that sucked bodies down, that constituted a second skin of earth difficult to escape, that brutalized bodies on a truly numbing scale, that lacerated skin with stunning efficiency, had the ironic effect of heightening the importance of intimate touches among men. The stunned, inured, desolate British soldier found maternal affirmation and warmth in the tactility of other men, an intimacy that was quite genuine. In the context of a modern war that proved so debilitating, soldiers caressed and held one another, kissed each other in an effort to come to terms with – and also escape – the twentieth century's first really radical expression of industrial modernity.[50]

The Artist's Touch

Even historians of sculpture – quite remarkably – have, according to Geraldine A. Johnson, "tended to overlook the question of touch in their studies." This sight-driven oversight is unfortunate, not least because it has impoverished our understanding of how central tactility was to ideas of beauty, knowledge, and meaning in the early modern period. Not only was sculpture considered at least as refined and intellectually vital as painting in early modern Italian culture (most famously, Michelangelo was obsessed with the power of the sculptor's generative touch), but sculpture facilitated a sort of interaction denied by two-dimensional art. For example, a sculpture remained, according to the Early Renaissance Florentine sculptor Lorenzo Ghiberti, inaccessible to sight, the eyes' sight merely glancing off the surface. True understanding and depth of meaning could come only through touch. So too long after the Renaissance. Bernard Berenson made a similar point with regard to painting in the 1890s. A painting, he maintained, must posses a tactile quality that touches and embraces the viewer for it to be excellent, and the art critic, Robert Hughes, has noted just such a propensity in John Constable's work.[51]

And while it is true that modern architecture and painting were heavily indebted to a Cartesian epistemology, it is also the case that some forms of visual expression attempted to promote hapticity over vision. Impressionism, for example, deliberately rejected perspectival depth and balanced framing (Cézanne hoped "to make visible how the world touches us"), while Cubists had no patience for a single focal point. Martin Jay offers similar arguments concerning the "baroque visual experience" that maintained "a strongly tactile or haptic quality, which prevents it from turning into the absolute ocularcentrism of its Cartesian perspectivalist rival." Of course, to claim that Cartesian perspective held an "absolute ocularcentrism" is too tidy, even clumsy, but it is nonetheless the case that the importance of the haptic was more than just an interesting sidelight to modernity. And there was good reason for the association between tactility and truth. As Ghiberti explained: "Touch only can discover [sculpture's] beauties which escape the sense of sight in any light." Such beliefs, while certainly diluted by the ocular-friendly Enlightenment, were never obliterated, living on as they did in a variety of ways.[52]

Lastly, it is worth mentioning in any discussion of art and tactility the importance of dance. If a visual-centered ballet was a product of the Renaissance, contact improvised dance, with its firm emphasis on the centrality of touch, was popular long after the widespread dissemination of print culture. Formally established in 1872 "when a group of Americans experimented with catching each other and falling together" and self-consciously opposed to the (perceived) ocularcentrism of ballet, contact improvisation is understood as a political statement, a form of dance that deliberately excludes sight: "Students often begin to learn contact improvisation by lying on the floor and closing their eyes, shutting off the stimulus of sight and thereby focusing more attentively on the skin of the whole body."[53]

Hapticity, Consumption, and Property

By way of conclusion to this chapter, I wish to pursue an important tactile thread running through the history of museums that grants us access to understanding the relationship between touch and ownership. The notion that touching equals possession is, as we have seen, deeply embedded in Western culture, as slaves in antiquity and during the nineteenth century, for example, well understood. This association was also very much alive even in nineteenth-century museums when patrons were urged to look at, but not touch, artifacts. As Constance Classen and David Howes have shown, although a resolutely visualist esthetic and practice percolated museums in the nineteenth and twentieth centuries, a process whereby "objects are colonized by the gaze," this had not always been the case and, in fact, was not always the case even at the height of modernity's championing of the eye. For example, visitors to Oxford's Ashmolean Museum in the early 1700s were allowed to hold artifacts and even though the Museum's curators were concerned that excessive handling might damage them, "they were unwilling to forbid such handling due to the notion that touch provided an essential – and expected – means of acquiring knowledge." Visitors to the British Museum in the 1780s fingered ashes in ancient urns and held objects to feel both the weight of the artifact and the past. Touch, for visitors, allowed them to engage in an imaginary conversation with the past, the tactile engagement firing their historical fantasies. Seeing alone was considered limiting because the eyes read only the surface of an object. Touch, conversely, was deemed an authenticator, a way to access truth. Objects that looked heavy could be, upon feeling, often light and hapticity was at times a more reliable guide to veracity than sight for museum visitors.[54]

In recent years, Western museums have actively encouraged visitors to experience their collections – or, rather, some parts of their collections – not just by looking but also by touching. According to Fiona Candlin, the (re)introduction of hapticity to the museum has been motivated not just by curatorial understanding of how visitors best understand the past (it seems that many visitors believe they get a better "feel" for the past by touching artifacts) but also by the dictates of government policy. Since funding for national museums is tied to audience statistics, there are real financial reasons to generate visitor numbers and allowing patrons to touch parts of collections has, it seems, helped increase the number of visitors to the ordinarily eye-oriented museum. Yet, as Candlin explains, there is something of a sleight of hand at work here in the invitation to handle: "interactive and sensory elements within museums form a way of negotiating and containing damage." Very rare objects are not touched, patrons do not have real choices over what they touch, and what they may touch serves to protect valuable items as much as it allows the handling of less valuable ones. At base, touch is still treated as a threat to objects rather than as a way to empower visitors' understanding of the past. Ownership still confers – and prohibits – the right to touch and even in ordinarily publicly funded museums, touch indicates commodity, property, and possession.[55]

In this respect, public institutions, such as museums, have surrendered tactility to the modern capitalist market place. While many museums have rejected and resisted meaningful engagement with tactility, some businesses have embraced it, principally as a way to invite and entice ownership. Both sites reaffirm the commodity-laden, property-riddled nature of tactility, of course, but modern consumption practices actively encourage touching as part of their logic. If you want to touch what you currently do not own go to a store, not a museum. For example, in its attempt to sell "nature," The Nature Company, a popular mall-based store in the United States, "sets products low on the shelves, often out of their boxes, inviting you to touch, experience." Likewise with Anheuser-Busch's Sea World experience which emphasizes not only sight but also the importance of tactile interaction with many of its attractions – hence the tag-line, "Touch the Magic." Touch seems as thoroughly implicated in modernity as sight and to tell the history of the key developments of the modern world without reference to hapticity is to remain blind to the importance of skin, tactility, and, ultimately, possession.[56]

Conclusion
Futures of Senses Past

It seems counterintuitive to offer a conclusion on a subject that is still very much in its infancy. For that reason, I'll "conclude" by doing no such thing. Instead, I'll offer two arguments – informed ruminations, if you will – concerning the nature of future work on sensory history.

The first argument offers a cautionary, methodological note. Precisely because sensory history is so alive and vibrant, we have yet to develop sustained and informed conversations about how best to understand and develop it. In this context, it is important to examine what seems to be an emerging debate among practitioners of sensory history between those historians – and no few museum curators – who think that the sensory recreation of the past is both possible and desirable and those who do not. Although the conversation is quite muted at present, it promises, I think, to become an important debate among sensory historians. Some scholars have begun to insist that sensory history should offer a usable past, to help history "live," and they have pondered not only how best to go about researching the senses but how best to present their findings to readers and miscellaneous audiences to achieve this goal. Other historians – and I'm among them – worry that such an approach comes close to offering an ahistorical understanding of the senses and suspect that the desire to "experience" the sensate past in this fashion tells us more about our modern conceits and attitudes toward consumption and the "use" of the past than it does about how people – and not "us" – experienced and attached meaning to sensory worlds.[1]

The second approach argues that we will not possess a full understanding of the evolution of the senses and the changing nature of sensory hierarchies until historians produce work that tackles all the senses – until, that is, they begin to emphasize intersensorality. This particular demand might well be a little premature since we still need a great deal of information on the history of individual senses – especially for smell, taste, and touch – for the premodern period generally, and for the non-West in all periods of history especially. (Part of my argument here is also to suggest specific areas in need of more research.) Yet this dearth should not serve to deflect attention from the way the senses worked together and the ways that contemporaries understood their articulation.

On Method

In his important recent book, *A History of the Senses*, Robert Jütte begins, quite rightly, by stressing the need to historicize the senses. He makes the case that historians especially are under some obligation "to distinguish between the historicity of a physical experience (in this case sense perception) and the form in which it has been preserved or handed down," that we "have to break with the aprioristic assumption of the 'naturalness' of sense perception." Or, as Constance Classen puts it: "the investigation of the sensory worlds of past eras should not merely describe the range of sounds and smells that existed at a particular time, as evocative as that might be, but should uncover the meanings those sounds and smells had for people."[2]

But historians, despite general nodded agreement on the importance of placing the senses in context, are, upon scrutiny, by no means in complete agreement on this important matter. As Jütte explains, some medical historians, such as Barbara Duden, have made the case that they especially must "break with the aprioristic assumption of the 'naturalness' of sense perception, which is a move that historians of medicine often find difficult to make, for they tend on the one hand to construe their object as the history of a problem or idea, and on the other hand to leave questions of 'natural history' to anthropologists or biologists."[3]

This problem – one best described as a quiet ahistorical epistemological tendency – is apparent in some recent work on sensory history. Take, for example, the important book on the sensory worlds of early America by Peter Charles Hoffer. In *Sensory Worlds of Early America*, Hoffer makes clear that "the very idea of the senses is a cultural convention", but he nevertheless posits sensory history as essentially a project in the recovery of a usable, consumable, experiential past. "Can we use our senses to replicate sensation in a world we have (almost) lost?" asks Hoffer. "I think the answer is yes," he says, "and perhaps more important, the project is worth the effort." He considers the argument that past actors "used their senses and perceived the world in a way so different from our own as to be unrecoverable now" little more than a "caveat," which should not deter us from developing a usable sensory past. "A sensory history should convey to the reader the feel of the past," Hoffer maintains, and he is convinced that we can "recover what others long ago saw, heard, and smelled."[4]

Hoffer's case is thoughtful. "If we assume also that we have the same perceptual apparatus as the people we are studying in the past, and can sense the world as they did," he argues, "we are another step closer to our objective," namely, experiencing the past the same way as "they" did. (Hoffer does not comment on the problematic nature of the universal "we" and "they".) Hoffer also calls for changes in the ways historians conduct research. Scholars "hunched for days over the flaking, yellowed pages of parchment rolls in the archives," are, he says, unlikely to "recapture that sensory past." Better to "follow children and their parents to the living museums that dot our country." He firmly believes that "living museums" and "commercial re-creations of the past and popular re-enactments" can "close the gap between then and now." "By engaging in sensory history we can stimulate our powers of imagination to their fullest extent," maintains Hoffer, "Such histories of the senses would fulfill the highest purpose of historical scholarship: to make the past live again" and, for Hoffer, living museums are important to that endeavor.[5]

Hoffer is far from alone here. Tourist and heritage industries make very similar claims. The "rediscovery of the senses has become a highly profitable business," argues Jütte and he points to not just the world of advertising but also living museums. "Canny exhibition curators," he explains, recognize the appeal of the sensory. While many of these museums attempt to convey something about the senses in contemporary culture, a couple have essayed to capture the history of the senses. An exhibition on food at the Hamburg Speicherstadtmuseum in 1999, for example, attempted to convey "the sensory experience of colonial produce that," according to Jütte, "had long lost its exotic character" by piping the smells of sugar, beer, wine, and tobacco "through a plastic tube fixed to the ceiling."[6]

There is nothing especially new about this. "Since the first organized Christmas celebration drew visitors to Colonial Williamsburg [Virginia] in 1936," visitors are told, "nothing quite matches the beauty, imagination, excitement, pageantry, sights, smells, sounds, and grandeur of the Christmas season in Colonial Williamsburg," a clever suggestion that what is experienced in the present is, in fact, a way to experience the past. The Colonial Williamsburg website happily invites us to "Experience the Life" of the eighteenth century and assures us that the "taste" of food served at various Williamsburg taverns is wholly "authentic," whatever that might mean.[7]

So, too, in Britain. In 1984, the York Archaeological Trust invited visitors to "Explore Viking history on the very site where archaeologists discovered the remains of the Viking city of Jorvik. Meet resident Vikings (staff), and see 800 of the items found during the dig. You can even journey back to a reconstruction of York in the year 975 CE, complete with the sights, sounds and smells of the Viking-Age!" The curators at Jorvik have managed to recreate – as they define it – the smells of the village, including the scent of the worryingly popular Viking latrine to which, we are told, visitors flock to get a healthy noseful, courtesy of scratch and sniff cards. Not only is this claim deeply misleading insofar as the smells Jorvik reproduces are necessarily wholly alien in meaning and content to the contemporary nose, but in the attempt to recreate the smell of a Viking village the curators necessarily add to the impression that the past was smellier than the present, thus cordoning off, in neat fashion, modernity as odorless and depicting premodernity as smelly. Rather than investigating the narrative that posits history becoming less olfactory as it progresses from a stench-ridden past, the Jorvik site simply reaffirms the conceit. But, as we have seen, smell was no less important to the modern era and claims about stench, smells, reeks were deeply implicated in any number of politically charged developments.[8]

The claims of places such as Colonial Williamsburg and Jorvik need to be taken seriously because they are, in fact, taken very seriously by many professionals, not least by some historians. Witness Dr. Wade Shaffer, associate professor of history at West Texas A&M University, who, in May 2005, took a group of students to Colonial Williamsburg to teach a course on colonial history. "There is nothing like being there to appreciate it," Shaffer said. "It always strikes me how few of our students have been to the east coast, where early American history took place. You can smell the history in places like Williamsburg, where the revolution virtually began, and Yorktown, where it ended in an American victory." He explains: "Your senses become heightened to where you can smell the gun powder... You see how people lived and learn what they felt was important. It's a fantastic way to teach a class or take one."[9] In other words, serious scholars and dedicated teachers, like Peter Hoffer and Wade Shaffer, argue a case for the desirability of a transcendent sensory past and their arguments should be taken seriously.

My principal objection to this argument is, simply put, that Hoffer and Shaffer and the curators/managers at Jorvik and Williamsburg – and, perhaps, the thousands of ardent re-enactors of the Civil War, too – wrongly marry the production of the past to its present-day consumption. Colonial Williamsburg claims that, for the price of admission, "history is alive every day."[10] The problem with all of this has to do with our apparent need to consume – and therefore render consumable – something which is, in fact, beyond consumption. While it is perfectly possible to recreate the decibel level and tone of a hammer hitting an anvil from the nineteenth century, or a piece of music from 1750 (especially if we still have the score and original instruments), or the taste of a given food from 1100, or the smell of dung from 1500 (I imagine that, chemically, the reproduction is feasible), it is impossible to experience those sensations the same way as those who heard the hammer or music, tasted the food, or smelled the dung. What was rank and fetid to, say, a tenth-century Viking's nostrils is not recoverable today, not least because that world – the world that shaped what smells existed and how they were perceived and understood by multiple constituencies – has evaporated. The same holds true for all historical evidence, visual and aural included. For example, "we" do not "see" the engraving of a slave whipping from the 1830s in the same light, with the same meaning, with the same emotional intensity or meaning as the abolitionist did at the time. That something as seemingly straightforward as a color – as Michel Pastoureau's wonderful history of the color blue makes clear – was, in fact, subject to significant variation not only in its meaning but in its very definition suggests the danger in making easy, ahistorical claims for the senses generally.[11]

Even the reproducibility of past sensations should not be taken for granted. Can we really recreate the sounds of eighteenth-century Williamsburg? What about the low rumble of jet planes overhead and the intrusive beat of nearby traffic? Should personal stereos be banned in such environments, lest degraded noise from earphones spill into the soundscape of those trying anxiously to experience the soundscape of Williamsburg "as it once was"? What of Civil War re-enactors in America? Can they really recreate battles in their full sensory texture? Acoustic shadows – accidents of climate and geography creating sounds that appeared to come from one direction but in reality emanated from another – were not unknown during Civil War engagements. Those conditions cannot be reproduced and so neither can the experience of those battles where acoustic shadows occurred be re-consumed, tempting though it can be to think otherwise.[12]

And when historians such as Hoffer write so enthusiastically about "us" and "we" are they really attending as carefully as they might to the context in which the senses worked? Even as Hoffer correctly stresses the importance of the plurality of the colonial American experience, rescuing the experience of African Americans, women, and Native Americans; even as he rightly calls for a carefully differentiated history, one that delineates the specific experiences of particular groups; even as he aims to take us beyond the U.S. nationalist narrative of the 1950s, he ends up replacing a nationalist sensory narrative with a universalist one in which "we," all of "us" in the present, can "experience" the past just as each, highly differentiated group did. In short, while it is possible to reproduce, for example, a particular sound from the eighteenth century it seems unlikely that visiting Williamsburg or Jorvik or any number of historical sites will explain how multiple constituencies (and not just "we") understood or consumed that same sound (or, indeed, noise).

That this argument over the historicity of the senses, their reproducibility, and whether or not we can (or ought) to try to re-experience the sensate past is beginning to have currency is surprising because it is not especially new. In his seminal commentary on how to best approach a history of the senses, Alain Corbin expressed reservations similar to the ones I outline here in his discussion of Guy Thuillier's "positivist" effort to "trace the evolution of the sensory environment." Thuillier, explained Corbin, "has attempted to compile a catalogue and measure the relative intensity of the noises which might reach the ear of a villager in the Nivernais in the middle of the nineteenth century." Indeed, there is something alluring about the apparent innocence of mere cataloging and even the best minds can be fooled. Even Corbin had some nice – if perhaps too charitable – things to say about this approach. He thinks that reading Thuiller's catalog "you can almost hear ... the ringing of the hammer on the anvil, the heavy thud of the wooden mallet wielded by the Cartwright, the insistent presence of bells and the whinny of horses in an aural environment where the noise of the amplifier was unknown." There are other reasons Corbin believes this approach "is by no means negligible": "It aids immersion in the village of the past; it encourages the adoption of a comprehensive viewpoint." But Corbin has thought too much and too carefully to endorse such thinking. Such an approach, he concludes, "is based on a questionable postulate, it implies the non-historicity of the modalities of attention, thresholds of perception, significance of noises, and configuration of the tolerable and the intolerable." Without a dedicated and careful attempt to attach meaning to those noises, cataloging is not only of very modest heuristic worth but, in fact, quite dangerous in its ability to inspire unwitting faith that these are the "real" sounds of the past.[13]

On Method – and Presentation

Hoffer's work (and the practices generally of some living museums and historic sites) raises not just phenomenological questions but closely related presentational ones. Asks Hoffer: "Even if historians can satisfy themselves that they can recover the sensory world of their ancestors, can they convey that sensory past to their auditors and readers?" Can sensory historians rely on print alone to accurately present their work to readers? Hoffer terms this the "lemon problem": "I can taste a lemon and savor the immediate experience of my senses; I can recall the taste after I have thrown away the fruit, but can I use words and pictures to fully understand what I am saying or, rather, to get at the reality behind my words?" Hoffer thinks we can reliably convey something of the taste of a lemon to readers.[14]

Imagine we could reproduce the taste of a lemon; that, courtesy of the gas liquid chromatographer (a machine able to reproduce flavors), Johns Hopkins University Press, which published Hoffer's book, reproduced a small square of lickable paper immediately following his paragraph about the taste of lemons. The reader simply licks the square and experiences what Hoffer experienced.

Or does he or she? How a lemon tastes is contingent on the tongue doing the licking, its specific history and culture. After all, cultural and historical specificity shapes all of the senses. Take, for example, the olfactory tastes of modern Britons and Americans – united by a common heritage, it seems, but separated by a different nose. Two studies – one performed in the 1960s in the U.K., the other a decade later in the U.S. – found that Britons disliked the smell of methyl salicylate (wintergreen) while Americans loved it. The problematical categories of "British" and "American" notwithstanding, historical specificity accounts for the learned preference. Among a particular generation in the U.K., the scent of wintergreen was associated with medicine and ointments used during the Second World War (not the best of times). Conversely, wintergreen in the U.S. is the olfactory cognate not of medicine but of candy (a minty smell). And this is just in the recent past. Imagine trying to recapture the "taste" of a particular food from, say, the fourteenth century when people who had yet to encounter sugar tasted in ways that would be different after sugar had been introduced to their diet. Thus, the taste of a lemon is far from historically or culturally constant and *how* it tastes, its meaning, its salivating sharpness or sweetness is dependent on many factors, the not least of which is history.[15]

That Hoffer should chose to illustrate his point with reference to the sense of taste is curious not least because historians and philosophers of taste especially have been sensitive to the historically conditioned meaning of how food tasted, perhaps because the field of inquiry necessarily engages the very ephemerality of the taste of food and drink and aesthetic judgment of taste, all of which sensitize scholars to the preeminent importance of context. As Carolyn Korsmeyer maintains: "acts of tasting occur within cultural contexts where eating traditions accustom people to a specific range of food and beverages." History is a key conditioner simply because cultures and societies "change as time passes, climate alters, societies undergo migration and colonization, and so forth. What people eat today is not the same as what they ate in the past, and one surmises that their taste worlds also differ." Thus, while we might engage in imaginative speculation about what a food tasted like to a certain group in the past, the authenticity and reproducibility of that taste to that particular constituency is beyond recovery.[16]

Philosopher Jean-François Revel offers a similar and, at times, quite stunning brief explaining why it is impossible to replicate flavors – and hence tastes – from the past. As he shows, not only are many foods no longer available but the traditions and contexts which gave those foods meaning and taste to a variety of constituencies makes it all but impossible to recreate and re-experience the taste. Revel applies a hard-nosed historicism to the question of taste, one that historians unduly enamored of the Williamsburgesque experience would do well to ponder carefully: "What did a meal, a wine *taste like* in the third century before or after Christ? And *what sort of taste* did the guests have?" It is, says Revel, impossible to know. Not only is habit everything when it comes to taste – and since habit is embedded and rarely defined explicitly, we cannot capture it from the past – but to "compound the difficulty of reconstructing what is remote from us, let us add that cuisine travels as badly in space as in time, and the same is true of information about cuisine." For example, the *paella valenciana* that is eaten in Valencia, he explains, "is based not on seafood but on rabbit." Certain foods and drinks not only no longer exist but contemporary descriptions of them – if they exist – as say, "sweet" or "dry," provide little guidance to those who hanker to recreate the taste of food in ancient Rome since the very definition of sweet and dry gastronomically is hostage to time and context and fundamentally non-exportable to the present. What is tasteful and what is tasteless is a product of context not least because the definitions of taste are frequently and actively defined by certain constituencies. Gastronomic literature in the nineteenth and twentieth centuries did not simply describe taste but, in the very process of narrating it, prescribed good taste and bad. Historians need to remain keenly vigilant that some of the narratives they use to reproduce an apparently antiseptic, pure understanding of taste in the past might actually be political sources with various kinds of authority lurking in the narratives themselves.[17]

In short, the idea that we can, at the point where historical sources stop, deploy our imaginations to capture and recreate tastes, is fictional not least because our capacity to imagine is heavily influenced by the values and context of the moment in time and place that we occupy. Moreover, print remains an effective medium for conveying the sensory meanings of the past. Through print, we can readily grasp what particular sensory events or stimuli meant to particular individuals and groups in particular contexts. If the print revolution did, in fact, elevate the eye and denigrate the nose, ear, tongue, and skin, printed evidence and the sensory perceptions recorded by contemporaries nevertheless constitute the principal medium through which we can access the senses of the past and their meanings.[18]

On Intersensoriality

It is no little irony that embedded within the great divide thesis – a thesis that this book has tried to qualify, a thesis that exaggerates the emergence of the eye and denigration of the other senses under modernity – is a keen insight that will likely shape the writing of sensory history for the foreseeable future. Even though McLuhan especially overstated the extent to which sight triumphed at the expense of the other senses by identifying a shift in the ratio of the senses, he nevertheless opened up analytic room for taking seriously the relationship among the senses. It is an insight that anthropologists and a few other scholars, including some art historians, have profitability taken up and one that historians should take more seriously. Historians are not alone here and David Howes has pointed out how "Western philosophers and psychologists have tended to treat the senses individually, ignoring the fact that they always act in concert." Given the initially modest amount of work on the history of the senses, relative to other topics, initial sense-specific forays into sensory history were understandable. Now, however, we are beginning to accumulate enough work for specific places and times – post-Revolutionary France and modern Europe generally, for example – where historians can profitably begin to think seriously about the interpretive value of examining how the senses worked together, sometimes in complimentary fashion, sometimes in tension.[19]

It might be most helpful to illustrate the benefits of historically informed intersensorial analysis – and, by, default, the limits of continuing to focus on just one sense – by way of example. A brief examination of the history of supermarkets in twentieth-century America is suggestive.

As many U.S. historians know, late Victorian department stores in the United States were very much influenced by a set of visual aesthetics, ones that tended to downplay the relevance of the other senses. Eye-catching, bright billboards and signs lured shoppers in and directed bright lighting focused their eyes on goods prominently displayed in glass cases. "Look but don't touch unless you'll buy," seemed to be the message. Here, department stores teased buyers through their eyes, heightening the anticipation of consumption by relying on visual displays.[20]

But after the Second World War, as historian Adam Mack has recently shown, American supermarkets went beyond the eyes. Certainly, supermarkets recognized the importance of lighting, brightness, and "eye appeal" in their stores, but they also, and increasingly, relied on the other senses to engage customers. Of course, seeing was still important, more so than ever in some respects, thanks largely to changes in technology. In the 1930s and 1940s, for example, merchants shifted from the indirect, yellow light of incandescent globes to more diffused, whiter, and revealing fluorescent lighting, creating something of a daylight effect inside stores. Large show windows also replaced small shop front windows so that what was inside could be clearly seen, especially from the vantage point of a car passenger. And what could be seen inside was increasingly the product of professional color engineers who used bright, pastel colors and combined them with hospital-clean white partly to suggest cleanliness but also to divorce the supermarket of the 1950s from the drab monotone associated with a colorless recession-era 1930s and war-time America.[21]

Such visual refinement went hand-in-hand with increasingly sophisticated reliance on the other senses and the modern American supermarket – how it worked, its meaning to contemporaries – cannot be understood fully outside this multisensory and intersensory context.

Increasing competition among American supermarkets after the Second World War and the standardization of goods that initially accompanied the emergence of the supermarket helped foster, in Mack's description, a "need for supermarkets that offered novelty, pleasure and fun," with carefully contrived and gender-specific "gustatory and erotic thrills" forming the basis of the modern American supermarket. Grocery retailers "turned to the sensual appeals of their merchandise, inviting customers to enjoy a range of sensory pleasures associated with food" and, in the process, invited customers, women especially, to indulge the pleasure of the sensate.[22]

For example, *Super Market Merchandising*, the industry trade journal, told managers in 1938: "There are only five ways in which a consumer can possibly be responsive to any selling appeal, namely through the senses of seeing, hearing, touching, tasting and smelling." Indeed, a good deal of what the journal counseled suggests why sensory history needs to embrace intersensoriality. Visual displays were intended to "hit 'em in the eye" and then the other senses would soothe and seduce customers once in the store, offering a sensorial "place of comfort and pleasure, as well as low prices."[23]

Intersensory joined multisensory approaches in post-war supermarket sales strategies. "Few customers can resist visibility of a product when combined with the added attraction of the sense of smell," reported *Chain Store Age* in 1956 when commenting on how best to peddle popcorn. The emergence of self-service was also important. "Before the rise of the supermarket," explains Mack, "food sellers had allowed buyers to handle their merchandise to a limited extent, typically to counter suspicions of spoilage or low quality. Supermarket companies, however, broke from the past because they encouraged consumers to handle, pinch and smell their fresh fruits and vegetables in the belief" that doing so would increase sales.[24]

And yet even as this multisensory strategy marked a break with the past in terms of how to sell food, it was also, quite deliberately, a play on historically framed sensory stereotypes. The association with women, the lower senses, and eroticism was obvious, unapologetic, and quite conscious, and supermarket pleasures were conceived of by managers as being similar to bazaars, markets, and marts of earlier times. Modern mass consumption in supermarkets specifically, then, owed something to the deliberate framing of taste as erotic, thus at once recalling and reinscribing a putatively age-old association between tongue and sex in a context devoted to the unapologetically modern, capitalist pursuit of profit. In other words, the sort of gustatory and tactile association used by supermarkets placed a premium on stressing a supposedly "premodern," sexually loaded and animal association of the senses of taste and touch.[25]

Not every sense operated this way in the modern supermarket and the aesthetics of sense changed over time, sometimes quite quickly. For example, by the end of the 1930s the days of boisterous markets were numbered. Instead, the silence of modernity reigned. Previously, when customers had been served in stores, sound, listening, talking, were important parts of the process of selling and buying. Self-service changed the soundscape of consumption and reconfigured what was deemed noise and what was considered sound in the context of buying. Absent the chatter and spoken world of actively engaged sales clerks, the modern supermarket turned the increasing necessity of silence into a virtue. A quieter supermarket, at least understood in terms of the spoken word, was considered desirable, a hallmark of efficiency, and aimed to attract a new, more middle-class customer base, one presumably more enamored of refined quietude than noisy, bazaar-like bustle. But scale generated noise. The customers, employees, cash registers, all were more numerous and so such noise was increasingly controlled by acoustic design, new sound-absorbing floors and ceilings that muffled sound, and registers and shopping carts that were touted as quiet and noiseless by their manufacturers. The modern shopping experience was supposed to be quiet, refined, and efficient.[26]

On the whole, then, the history of supermarkets in twentieth-century America suggests not only the benefits but also the need for sensory history to pay greater attention to multi- and intersensorality. To examine just the role of sound in this history, for example, would warp understanding and suggest that supermarkets not only did not deploy other sensory strategies to prime consumption but that they were not interested in the use – and continued construction – of putatively premodern senses, such as taste, touch, and smell. Here, the example of intersensorality suggests how impoverished an understanding that cleaves too literally to the great divide theory can be. Instead, recognizing the function and importance of multiple senses, and how they might have operated in concert (or even in tension), illustrates how supposedly premodern senses proved fugitive and were imported into modernity. It makes better sense to recognize that the empowerment of the eye did not work in a zero-sum fashion. The other senses not only remained important, they became critical to modernity, a point made especially clear when we consider the ways in which the senses functioned together.

Possible Futures

A fuller understanding of sensory history can be achieved only with more work on a number of areas, especially for the premodern period and particularly for the non-West for all eras. But even for the modern period generally, which is arguably the best-represented in the literature, we lack research on dozens of topics. We could, for example, profitably explore in much greater detail the sensory worlds of children, not least because, as with most historical inquiry, it is the experience of adults that sensory history has taken most seriously. But children might well have understood the senses differently because they were often in the process of learning the social protocols and cultural expectations of their society with regard to the meaning and value of the various senses. We also need research especially in fields that at first blush seem barren soil for sensory history, fields of inquiry that some might consider old fashioned and hostage to a particular way of understanding the past that seem to offer little room for serious work on the senses. Here, I will offer just two examples.

The first concerns historical biography – a field of inquiry frequently so heavy on the study of politics that the senses would seem to have little room to flourish. And yet, as Sander Gilman has rightly suggested, we can profitability approach the history of individuals and write historical biographies using sensory history. Gilman argued in his fascinating study of Johann Wolfgang von Goethe and tactility that while the "idea of a social history of the senses has come of age," much of that work has operated from the "assumption ... that the history of *all* of the senses could be written as part of the history of the *mentalité*, the historically created consciousness of any given culture." Why not, asked Gilman, also try to "understand how central individual variations are in shaping the generalized response of a culture"? There are dangers with such an approach, of course. Depending on the subject under consideration, a sensory biography might quickly become an interior intellectual history project that does not deal with the senses in a fully textured or articulated way. The second danger is that a foray into sensory biography might wrongly posit the social and cultural history of the senses and sensory biography as somehow in tension when, in fact, the tools and insights of social history could be used when detailing how any given individual understood the senses and the context in which he or she lived. Gilman comes perilously near to endorsing such a position when he says that "it is not the general setting but the specific individual response, with all its personal idiosyncrasies, that is of real interest in writing a history of the senses." This distinction is both unhelpful and false not least because one cannot measure idiosyncratic sensory understanding without having an understanding of the general sensescape of a society and culture. Such caveats in mind, it does seem helpful to turn to biographical treatments and bring sensory history to bear on especially complicated historical figures whose behavior and reasons for acting in a particular way in a certain context might be better understood by attending less to what he or she saw of the world and more to what he or she felt, or smelled, or heard, or tasted.[27]

A second field that might attract the attention of sensory historians and that might adopt some of the habits of sensory history is diplomatic history. In fact, a few diplomatic historians have begun to take the senses seriously and have paid particular attention to how sensory stereotypes allow us to understand better the construction of the other that frequently guides in quiet but meaningful ways official foreign policies. This development could prove very helpful to students not only of "foreign" affairs but to scholars who understand that a country's foreign policy and the cultural values that drive it – including sensory ones – reveals as much about domestic polices as foreign ones. Certainly, such initiatives could profitably build on the growing body of work relating the senses to the emergence of the nation-state, nationalism, and ethnicity (some of it detailed in this book). For example, as Andrew J. Rotter in his fascinating study of U.S.–India relations in the twentieth century has shown, Asia generally, India in particular, was smelled as much as seen in Western minds. In part because Americans especially found India "inscrutable," hidden by a "veil" that prevented them from "seeing its features clearly," they found their "truths" about India less in the eye and more in the nose. In some early Western estimations, some Indians had no mouths and "live[d] on the smell of roast beef and the odors of flowers and fruit." Later olfactory stereotypes associated India with the smell of feces, "the land of shit," and indexed the smell of open sewers with ideas about a barbaric, uncivilized state. Such associations proved especially troubling, argues Rotter, not least because the smell of feces and what it meant reminded Americans "who they had been and who they might still be." Future studies of diplomatic histories, provided they become attuned to the sensate, might well find smell and taste especially – frequently the senses most associated with a national identity – occupying important ground in the way that foreign affairs were conducted by powerful and weaker nation-states. The main challenge in pursuing this line of inquiry is to identify precisely how boarder cultural conceits about the senses and "foreigners" fed into the often terse and "diplomatic" discourse that, by its very nature, tended not to make obvious statements about smelly foreigners and the like, at least not in publicly released documents in the modern era.[28]

In both instances, and, in fact, whenever historians attend to the history of the senses, not only should they try to historicize and contextualize the senses but they might also attend to the importance of sensory metaphor. Taking seriously historically situated sensory metaphors is important because understanding how contemporaries used and invented sensory metaphors thoroughly complicates the notion of "proximate" senses. Through metaphor, smells, tastes, touches, and sounds broke free of their physical space, slipping into wide social and cultural circulation. In this way, the construction of, for example, sensory otherness became independent of immediate interaction and physical encounter. By way of illustration: the notion that black people had a distinctive odor gained national currency in both the nineteenth- and twentieth-century U.S., even though many people who believed the stereotype had virtually no direct contact with African Americans. And when whites did encounter African Americans the stereotype, already in place and of metaphoric status, predisposed them to believe that black people did, in fact, smell, even though, obviously, no such racial odor exists. A similar conceit and sensory mechanism was at work for many immigrant communities and also globally, with sensory stereotypes migrating beyond the borders of the nation-state. Printed words did not always stabilize vision and it is important to recognize how print itself served to empower, through metaphor and description, the non-visual senses granting them the ability to reach audiences far removed in space and time.[29]

More, much more, could be said, of course, but I will leave those contributions to others. For the moment, it seems enough to say that sensory history is full of potential, holds genuinely inter- and intra-disciplinary promise, and could prove to be of enduring importance. The real contribution of sensory history, though, might, ironically enough, best be measured in its dilution, evaporation, and reconfiguration. If, over the coming decades, sensory historians generally begin to include all of the senses in their studies, they could hope that their habit of attending to the sensate will begin to percolate into the profession at large and into the general writing of history in the form of sustained, serious, and explicit attention not just to sight but also to hearing, smelling, tasting, and touching in the writing and conceptualization of history generally. Until that time, however, sensory historians are very much obliged to keep making their case, keep producing their work, and keep attending to the importance of the senses in the history of human experience.

Notes

Introduction

1. See Penelope Gouk, "Raising Spirits and Restoring Souls: Early Modern Medical Explanations for Music's Effects," in Viet Erlmann (ed.), *Hearing Cultures: Essays on Sound, Listening and Modernity* (Oxford: Berg, 2004), p. 87.

2. I happily recognize the importance of all sorts of subfields to social history's larger project of capturing the history of the sensate in my essay "Making Sense of Social History." For my purposes here, I use the terms social and cultural history as an umbrella under which I gather any number of other subfields such as environmental history, the history of technology, the history of medicine, histories of structures and values generally, to identify just a few.

3. Constance Classen, "Foundations for an Anthropology of the Senses," *International Social Science Journal* 153 (September 1997), p. 401 (first quotation); Constance Classen, *Worlds of Sense: Exploring the Senses in History and Across Cultures* (New York: Routledge, 1993), p. 1 (second quotation). See also the thoughtful remarks in Michel Pastoureau, *Blue: The History of a Color* (Princeton, NJ: Princeton University Press, 2001), pp. 7–10 esp. For an emphasis on the importance of cultural context for understanding the senses, see Kathryn Linn Geurts, *Culture and the Senses: Bodily Ways of Knowing in an African Community* (Berkeley: University of California Press, 2002). Piero Camporesi's study, *The Anatomy of the Senses: Natural Symbols in Medieval and Early Modern Italy*, Allan Cameron (trans.) (Cambridge: Polity Press, 1994), tends toward a sensuous reading of history, as Constance Classen points out in "The Senses," in Peter N. Stearns (ed.), *Encyclopedia of European Social History From 1350–2000*, 4 (New York: Gale, 2001), p. 357. A popular book that does not historicize the senses is Diane Ackerman's *A Natural History of the Senses* (New York: Vintage, 1991).

4. I am less interested in the history of how Western societies especially came to endorse the idea that there are five senses rather than, say, seven or eight. As Classen explains: "Culture shapes the senses in many ways. The number of the senses is dictated to some extent by custom. While the senses are generally counted as five – sight, hearing, smell, taste, and touch – their number has risen

or fallen at different times according to the interests of the day." Suffice to say, the number of senses was subject to some debate and very much a product of prevailing religious and scientific ideologies. Classen, "The Senses," p. 355; Robert Rivlin and Karen Gravelle, *Deciphering the Senses: The Expanding World of Human Perception* (New York: Simon and Schuster, 1985), p. 15.

5. Robert Jütte refers to the history of sense perception. See his *A History of the Senses: From Antiquity to Cyberspace*, James Lynn (trans.) (Cambridge: Polity Press, 2005), p. 13. On historians' tendency to privilege the ocular, much has been written. See especially Martin Jay, *Downcast Eyes: The Denigration of Vision in Twentieth-Century French Thought* (Berkeley: University of California Press, 1993), pp. 45, 66–69; Classen, *Worlds of Sense*; George H. Roeder, Jr, "Coming to Our Senses," *Journal of American History* 81 (December 1994), p. 1114; see also my "Listening Back," in Mark M. Smith (ed.), *Hearing History: A Reader* (Athens, GA: University of Georgia Press, 2004), pp. 398–401.

6. Jütte, *History of the Senses*, p. 1. And, as anthropologist David Howes has made clear, neither should we necessarily assume that the postmodern, linguistic turn has been pivotal in generating interest in the senses. In fact, postmodern ethnography might well have anaesthetized some scholars against the sensory, privileging as it does writing, text, script, and vision. More than a mere expansion of "social science discourse on the body so as to include the senses," sensory history works to examine the senses qua senses and it is worth remembering – and re-reading – some older works that attended to the senses in imaginative and creative ways. See David Howes, "Introduction: 'To Summon All the Senses'," in David Howes (ed.), *Sensual Relations: Engaging the Senses in Culture and Social Theory* (Ann Arbor: University of Michigan Press, 2003), p. 4; Howes *Sensual Relations: Engaging the Senses in Culture and Social Theory* (Ann Arbor: University of Michigan Press, 2003), p. xii; Howes, "Controlling Textuality: A Call for a Return to the Senses," *Anthropologica* 33 (1990), pp. 55–56; Stoller, *Sensuous Scholarship* (Philadelphia: University of Pennsylvania Press, 1997), pp. ix–xviii. For a geographer who stresses the importance of the work of postmodern theorists for alerting his profession to the senses, see Sui, "Visuality, Aurality, and Shifting Metaphors of Geographical Thought in the Late Twentieth Century," *Annals of the Association of American Geographers* 90 (2000), pp. 325–328. Sensory history has become quite public of late, with high-profile pieces featured in the *New York Times* (Emily Eakin, "History You Can See, Hear, Smell, Touch, and Taste," Saturday, December 20, 2003), the *Australian Review of Books* (Douglas Kahn, "Sound Awake," July 2000), and the recent and highly innovative series on the history of the senses on Chicago Public Radio's "Odyssey," hosted by Gretchen Helfrich, which aired in May and June in 2005. Recordings for each session are on line at http://www.wbez.org/programs/odyssey/odyssey_senses.asp. For a helpful overview of current interest in the senses, measured by the number of international conferences on the topic in recent years and the proliferation of scholarly work across disciplines, see Howes, "Forming Perceptions," in

David Howes (ed.) *Empire of the Senses: The Sensual Culture Reader* (Oxford: Berg, 2005), pp. 399–402.

7. Lucien Febvre, *The Problem of Unbelief in the Sixteenth Century: The Religion of Rabelais*, Beatrice Gottlieb (trans.) (Cambridge, MA: Harvard University Press, 1982), pp. 11, 12.

8. Leigh Eric Schmidt, *Hearing Things: Religion, Illusions, and the American Enlightenment* (Cambridge, MA: Harvard University Press, 2000), p. 18.

9. Michel Foucault, *The Order of Things: An Archaeology of the Human Sciences* (New York: Vintage Books, 1994), p. 132; Michel Foucault, *The Birth of the Clinic: An Archaeology of Medical Perception*, A. M. Sheridan Smith (trans.) (New York: Vintage Books, 1975; David Howes and Marc Lalonde, "The History of Sensibilities: Of the Standard of Taste In Mid-Eighteenth Century England and the Circulation of Smells in Post-Revolutionary France," *Dialectical Anthropology* 16 (1991), p. 132.

10. Alain Corbin, *The Foul and the Fragrant: Odor and the French Social Imagination*, Miriam Kochan, Roy Porter, and Christopher Prendergast (trans.) (Cambridge, MA: Harvard University Press, 1986); Corbin, *Time, Desire and Horror: Towards a History of the Senses*, Jean Birrell (trans.) (Cambridge: Polity Press, 1995); Corbin, *Village Bells: Sound and Meaning in the 19th-Century French Countryside*, Martin Thom (trans.) (New York: Columbia University Press, 1998); Sima Godfrey, "Alain Corbin: Making Sense of French History," *French Historical Studies*, 25 (Spring 2002); Corbin, *Time, Desire and Horror*, 181–182, 183. See also Schmidt, *Hearing Things*, 18; Mark M. Smith, "Making Sense of Social History," *Journal of Social History* 37 (Fall 2003), pp. 165–186. Anthropologists have been at the forefront of establishing the importance of sensory experience and some of the most theoretically sophisticated practitioners have been engaged in the project since at least the 1970s. Sensory history owes a great deal to their work. On the importance of anthropologists to the scholarly investigation of the senses, see Howes, *Sensual Relations*, p. xiii; David Howes (ed.), *The Varieties of Sensory Experience: A Sourcebook in the Anthropology of the Senses* (Toronto: University of Toronto Press, 1991). For related work by geographers, see Paul Rodaway, *Sensuous Geographies: Body, Sense and Place* (London: Routledge, 1994); Pocock, "The Senses in Focus," in W. F. Bynum and Roy Porter (eds), *Medicine and the Five Senses* (Cambridge: Cambridge University Press, 1993), pp. 11–16; Daniel Z. Sui, "Visuality, Aurality, and Shifting Metaphors," *Annals of the Association of American Geographers* 90 (2000), pp. 322–343; Susan J. Smith, "Beyond Geography's Visible Worlds: A Cultural Politics of Music," *Progress in Human Geography* 21 (1997). Historians generally have been a little slower on the sensory uptake and some of those who have begun to take the senses seriously, myself included, have been influenced by the pioneering work of anthropologists. To be fair, some historians, particularly those who study European history and especially those working in Canadian institutions, have been especially attentive to sensory history. Historians John E. Crowley and Joy Parr and anthropologists Constance Classen, David Howes, and Anthony

Synnott have written thoughtfully and innovatively on aspects of the history of the senses. Why the intellectual and programmatic interest in the senses at Canadian universities is unclear but it might have something to do with the early work on sound and the senses by R. Murray Schafer and Barry Truax (both of the World Soundscape Project at Simon Fraser University), and, even earlier, Harold Innis and Marshall McLuhan, among others. On this Canadian influence, see Joy Parr, "Notes for a More Sensuous History of Twentieth-Century Canada: The Timely, the Tacit, and the Material Body," *Canadian Historical Review* 82 (December 2001)," pp. 733, n.36.

11. W. F. Bynum and Roy Porter, "Introduction," in *Medicine and the Fine Senses* (Cambridge: Cambridge University Press, 1993), pp. 1–2. Corbin's analysis in *Time, Desire, Horror* is also heavily indented to an understanding of public health.

12. Lisa Gitelman, *Scripts, Grooves, and Writing Machines: Representing Technology in the Edison Era* (Stanford, CA: Stanford University Press, 1999); Jonathan Sterne, *The Audible Past: Cultural Origins of Sound Reproduction* (Durham, NC: Duke University Press, 2003); Emily Thompson, *The Soundscape of Modernity: Architectural Acoustics and the Culture of Listening in America, 1900–1933* (Cambridge, MA: MIT Press, 2002); Douglas Kahn, *Noise, Water, Meat: A History of Sound in the Arts* (Cambridge, MA: MIT Press, 1999) approach the topic by way of communication and media studies, the history of technology, and art history. Legal historians have written a fair bit on the senses. See most obviously the essays in Lionel Bently and Leo Flynn (eds), *Law and the Senses Senses: Sensational Jurisprudence* (London: Pluto Press, 1996); Bernard J. Hibbitts, "Making Sense of Metaphors"; Hibbitts, "Coming to Our Senses: Communication and Legal Expression in Performance Culture" 41 *Emory Law Journal* 4 (1992), pp. 874–959. Environmental historians have been especially sensitive to questions of sensory experience. As early as the 1970s, for example, Raymond W. Smilor produced important work on noise. See his "Cacophony at 34th and 6th: The Noise Problem in America, 1900–1930," *American Studies*, 18 (1977), pp. 23–38, "Confronting the Industrial Environment: The Noise Problem in America, 1893–1932," Ph.D. dissertation, University of Texas, 1978, and "Personal Boundaries in the Urban Environment: The Legal Attack on Noise: 1865–1930," *Environmental Review*, 3 (1979). Peter A. Coates has recently taken up where Smilor left off. See his "The Strange Stillness of the Past: Toward an Environmental History of Sound and Noise," *Environmental History* 10 (October 2005). Note also Sima Godfrey, "Alain Corbin: Making Sense of French History," *French Historical Studies*, 25 (Spring 2002), p. 387. For a braiding of environmental, business, and legal history, see Christine Rosen, "'Knowing' Industrial Pollution: Nuisance Law and the Power of Tradition in a Time of Rapid Economic Change, 1840–1864," *Environmental History* 8 (October 2003). On how work by feminist scholars has furthered our understanding of the gendering of the senses, see Constance Classen, "The Senses," in Peter N. Stearns (ed.), *Encyclopedia of European Social History From 1350–2000*, 4 (New

York: Gale, 2001), p. 358. Historians and scholars of religion especially, perhaps because of the historical importance of the spiritual senses and the sensory dimensions to faith and knowing, have produced some deeply thoughtful work on the senses. See, especially, Leigh Schmidt, *Hearing Things: Religion, Illusions, and the American Enlightenment* (Cambridge, MA: Harvard University Press, 2000); David Chidester, *Word and Light: Seeing, Hearing, and Religious Discourse* (Urbana: University of Illinois Press, 1992); Chidester, "The American Touch: Tactile Imagery in American Religion and Politics," in Constance Classen (ed.), *The Book of Touch* (Oxford: Berg, 2005); Susan Ashbrook Harvey, *Scenting Salvation: Ancient Christianity and the Olfactory Imagination* (Berkeley: University of California Press, 2006), among others. On urban history, see particularly Jill Steward and Alexander Cowan (eds), *The City and the Senses: Urban Culture Since 1550* (Aldershot: Ashgate, 2007).

13. George H. Roeder, Jr., "Coming to our Senses," *Journal of American History* 81 (December 1994) pp. 1112–1113.

14. David Howes, "Sensorial Anthropology," in David Howes (ed.), *The Varieties of Sensory Experience: A Sourcebook in the Anthropology of the Senses* (Toronto: University of Toronto Press, 1991), p. 70.

15. Howes, "Sensorial Anthropology," pp. 170, 172; Marshall McLuhan, *The Gutenberg Galaxy* (Toronto: University of Toronto Press, 1962), pp. 28, 159–160, quotation on reading in the Middle Ages from Dom Jean Leclerq on p. 89; Walter J. Ong, *Orality and Literacy: The Technologizing of the Word* (New York: Routledge, 1982), pp. 72–73; McLuhan, *Understanding Media: The Extensions of Man* (Cambridge, MA: MIT Press, 1994 [1964]), pp. 265–270.

16. McLuhan, *The Gutenberg Galaxy*, pp. 159–160; McLuhan, *Understanding Media*, pp. 263–269. For a recent restatement of much of the great divide thesis, see Hibbitts, "Coming to Our Senses," [1.7–1.8] (reference is to the on-line version and indicates paragraph numbers). Note, too, Jack Goody, *The Logic of Writing and the Organization of Society* (Cambridge: Cambridge University Press, 1986); Goody, *The Interface between the Written and the Oral* (Cambridge: Cambridge University Press, 1987).

17. Howes, "Introduction: 'To Summon All the Senses'," pp. 11–14.

18. Howes, "Introduction: 'To Summon All the Senses'," pp. 12–13; Walter Ong, *The Presence of the Word* (New Haven, CT: Yale University Press, 1967); Ong, "The Shifting Sensorium," in David Howes (ed.), *The Varieties of Sensory Experience: A Sourcebook in the Anthropology of the Senses* (Toronto: University of Toronto Press, 1991), pp. 29–30; Ong, *Orality and Literacy*, p. 117.

19. Howes, "Introduction: 'To Summon All the Senses'," p. 8. The corollary to the McLuhan thesis – that non-Western societies are, by default, more attuned to non-visual senses – has received considerable support from scholars in other disciplines. Some social psychologists, for example, found that West African cultures "contain considerable emphasis on sensory phenomena apart from the visual world" and that only with the arrival of print was their principally auditory and tactile world rendered more ocular. See Mallory Wober,

"Sensotypes," *Journal of Social Psychology* 70 (October 1966), p. 182 (quotation), pp. 187–188.

20. McLuhan, *Gutenberg Galaxy*, p. 27.

21. Hibbitts, "Coming to Our Senses," [1.3, 4.1, 4.2].

22. Quotations, in order: Howes, "Sensorial Anthropology," p. 173; Classen, "The Senses," pp. 358–359; Classen, *Worlds of Sense*, p. 50. More recently, though, some anthropologists have suggested that orality theory does not stand up to scrutiny for a number of largely preliterate societies. Howes, for example, has shown how very visual some Papua New Guinea societies are, especially with regard to art, even though they are often non-literate, a condition that, according to McLuhan and Ong, should render them largely aural societies. They are not. Howes, *Sensual Relations*, chs. 4–6.

23. Schmidt, *Hearing Things*, pp. 7–8, 19–21, 22.

24. Jütte, *History of the Senses*, pp. 15, 16.

25. Stewart, "Prologue: From the Museum of Touch," in Marius Kwint, Christopher Breward, and Jeremy Aynsley (eds), *Material Memories* (Oxford: Berg, 1999), pp. 17, 19, 23; Corbin, *Time, Desire, Horror*, p. 190. For thoughtful and suggestive remarks on the ocularcentrism of modern academics in particular, see Constance Classen *The Book of Touch* (Oxford: Berg, 2005), p. 5. On Marx, note Jütte, *History of the Senses*, pp. 9–10. For a deeply learned – and compelling – examination of the protracted nature of the print revolution (which took almost four centuries), see David McKitterick, *Print, Manuscript and the Search for Order 1450–1830* (Cambridge: Cambridge University Press, 2003). On French intellectual discourse, see Martin Jay, *Downcast Eyes: The Denigration of Vision in Twentieth-Century French Thought* (Berkeley: University of California Press, 1993), p. 15 esp.

26. Corbin, *Time, Desire, Horror*, pp. 186–187.

27. I share some of Martin Jay's reservations about positing a wholly visualist "modern" against an anti-visuality premodern or Middle Ages. See Jay, *Downcast Eyes*, pp. 34–35, 41, and Schmidt, *Hearing Things*, p. 18.

28. Classen, "The Senses," p. 358. Classen also does a fine job of bringing into dialogue social and intellectual history in *The Color of Angels: Cosmology, Gender and the Aesthetic Imagination* (New York: Routledge, 1998).

29. Hunt, *Governance of the Consuming Passions: A History of Sumptuary Law* (New York: St. Martin's Press, 1996), pp. 12, x, xviii.

30. See especially Howes, "Introduction: 'To Summon All the Senses'," p. 17. In general, I am in sympathy with Carolyn Korsmeyer's brief but astute observation that the "presence of diverse opinion within the writings of Western philosophy – or any intellectual tradition – are important to bear in mind, for it is all too easy to obscure complexity and subtlety with sweeping generalizations." Korsmeyer's comment refers principally to the history of taste but it applies equally well to our understanding of the senses generally. Korsmeyer, "Introduction: Perspectives on Tastes," in Carolyn Korsmeyer (ed.), *The Taste Culture Reader: Experiencing Food and Drink* (Oxford: Berg, 2005), p. 2.

31. Mark Jenner, "Civilization and Deodorization? Smell in Early Modern English Culture," in Peter Burke, Brian Harrison, and Paul Slack (eds), *Civil Histories: Essays Presented to Sir Keith Thomas* (New York: Oxford University Press, 2000), pp. 129–130 (quotation), 130, 143–144.

32. While it is certainly true, as Jim Drobnick has argued, that vision has a "deep complicity with the subjugating forces of capitalism, colonialism and patriarchy" – modernity, in short – it is also the case that the non-visual senses were also deeply implicated in the multiple iterations of modernity. Drobnick, "Reveries, Assaults and Evaporating Presences: Olfactory Dimensions in Contemporary Art," *Parachute* 89 (1998), p. 10. Note, too, David Howes, "Scent and Sensibility," *Culture, Medicine and Psychiatry* 13 (1989); Howes and Lalonde, "The History of Sensibilities," p. 126.

Chapter 1 Look Here: Seeing the Light

1. Howes, *Sensual Relations*, pp. xii, xiii. On ocularcentrism, see Jay, *Downcast Eyes*, pp. 3, 21–82, 522–524; David Levin (ed.), *Modernity and the Hegemony of Vision* (Berkeley: University of California Press, 1993); Elliot Wolfson, *Through a Speculum That Shines: Vision and Imagination in Medieval Jewish Mysticism* (Princeton, NJ: Princeton University Press, 1994), p. 5; Luce Irigaray, *Speculum of the Other Woman*, Gillian C. Hill (trans.) (Ithaca, NY: Cornell University Press, 1985), pp. 46–48; Hans Jonas, "The Nobility of Sight: A Study in the Phenomenology of the Senses," in *The Phenomenon of Life: Toward a Philosophical Biology* (New York: Harper and Row, 1966).

2. Jay, *Downcast Eyes*, pp. 45, 66–69. See, also, the helpful critiques in: Constance Classen, *Worlds of Sense: Exploring the Senses in History and Across Cultures* (New York: Routledge, 1993); Jonathan Crary, *Techniques of the Observer: On Vision and Modernity in the Nineteenth Century* (Cambridge, MA: MIT Press, 1992); Kate Flint, *The Victorians and the Visual Imagination* (New York: Cambridge University Press, 2000); and Randolph Starn, "Seeing Culture in a Room for a Renaissance Prince," in Lynn Hunt (ed.), *The New Cultural History* (Berkeley: University of California Press, 1989), pp. 205–232. For an art historian who questions the centrality and authority of vision, see James Elkins, *The Object Stares Back: On the Nature of Seeing* (San Diego: Harvest, 1996); Elkins, *Visual Studies: A Skeptical Introduction* (New York: Routledge, 2003). Note, too, the influential work of John Berger, *Ways of Seeing* (London: Penguin, 1972). A recent and immensely thoughtful collection of essays is in Deborah Cherry (ed.), *Art: History: Visual: Culture* (Malden, MA: Blackwell, 2005).

3. Steven Connor, "The Modern Auditory I," in Roy Porter (ed.), *Rewriting the Self: Histories from the Renaissance to the Present* (London: Routledge, 1997), pp. 203–223.

4. Connor quoted in Mark M. Smith, (ed.), *Hearing History: A Reader* (Athens, GA: University of Georgia Press, 2004), pp. xiii–xiv.

5. Constance Classen and David Howes, "The Museum as Sensescape: Western Sensibilities and Indigenous Artefacts," in Elizabeth Edwards, Chris Gosden, and Ruth Phillips (eds), *Sensible Objects: Colonialism, Museums and Material Culture* (Oxford: Berg, 2006), pp. 199–222.

6. Donald Lowe, *History of Bourgeois Perception* (Chicago: University of Chicago Press, 1982), p. 13; Levin, *Modernity and the Hegemony of Vision*, pp. 2, 212; Hibbitts, Bernard J., "Coming to Our Senses" pp. 874–959, [3.15].

7. Murray Schafer, *The Soundscape: Our Sonic Environment and the Tuning of the World* (Rochester, VT: Inner Traditions, 1994), pp. 3–12.

8. Richard Rath, *How Early America Sounded* (Ithaca, NY: Cornell University Press, 2003), pp. 174, 177–178.

9. Howes, "Introduction: 'To Summon All the Senses'," p. 5; Parr, "Notes for a More Sensuous History of Twentieth-Century Canada," p. 736; Constance Classen, "Foundations for an Anthropology of the Senses," *International Social Science Journal* 153 (September 1997), p. 402; Informant 9F, "Russian Sensory Images," in Margaret Mead and Rhoda Métraux (eds), *The Study of Culture at a Distance* (Chicago: University of Chicago Press, 1953), p. 168. Some historians of architecture also detect what they term modernity's tendency toward retinal architecture, the loss of plasticity, and the "suppression of the other senses by means of technological extensions of the eye." Since Alberti, Western architecture, explains Juhani Pallasmaa, has been "engaged primarily with questions of visual perception, harmony and proportion," one captured by Alberti's statement that "Painting is nothing but the intersection of the visual pyramid following a given distance, a fixed centre and certain lighting," see Juhani Pallasmaa, *The Eyes of the Skin: Architecture and the Senses* (London: Academy Editions, 1996), pp. 16, 17.

10. Cynthia Cohen Bull, "Sense, Meaning, and Perception in Three Dance Cultures," in Jane C. Desmond (ed.) *Meaning in Motion: New Cultural Studies of Dance* (Durham, NC: Duke University Press, 1997), pp. 272 (quotation), 274.

11. Quoted in Classen and Howes, "The Museum as Sensescape," p. 199.

12. See Valentine Daniel, "The Pulse as an Icon in Siddha Medicine," in David Howes (ed.), *The Varieties of Sensory Experience: A Sourcebook in the Anthropology of the Senses* (Toronto: University of Toronto Press, 1991), pp. 107–108.

13. Classen, "The Senses," p. 361.

14. Classen, "The Senses," p. 361; Corbin, *Time, Desire and Horror: Towards a History of the Senses*, p. viii.

15. Michel Foucault, *Discipline and Punish: The Birth of the Prison*, Alan Sheridan (trans.) (New York: Penguin, 1987), pp. 200, 201. See also Crary, *Techniques of the Observer*, pp. 17–18; Michel Meranze, "Michel Foucault, the Death Penalty and the Crisis of Historical Understanding," *Historical Reflections/Réflexions Historiques* 29 (2003), pp. 202–203 esp.

16. M. J. Bouman, "The 'good lamp is the best police' metaphor and ideologies of the nineteenth-century urban landscape," *American Studies*, 32

(1991), pp. 63–78; Bouman, "Luxury and control: the urbanity of street lighting in nineteenth-century cities," *Journal of Urban History* 14 (1987), pp. 7–37; Samuel Martland, "Constructing Valparaiso: Infrastructure and the Politics of Progress in Chile's Port, 1842–1918," Ph.D. dissertation, University of Illinois at Urbana-Champaign, 2003; Wolfgang Schivelbusch, *Disenchanted Night: The Industrialization of Light in the Nineteenth Century* (Berkeley: University of California Press, 1988).

17. Classen, "The Senses," p. 362; Corbin, *Time, Desire, Horror*, p. ix; Roger Smith, "Self-Reflection and the Self," in Roy Porter (ed.), *Rewriting the Self: Histories from the Renaissance to the Present* (London and New York: Routledge, 1997), pp. 52–53.

18. Ong, *The Presence of the Word*, p. 74; Classen, *Worlds of Sense*, p. 16; Mark M. Smith, *How Race Is Made: Slavery, Segregation, and the Senses* (Chapel Hill: University of North Carolina Press, 2006), pp. 66–95.

19. Hibbitts, "Coming to Our Senses," [2.25]; Pallasmaa, *The Eyes of the Skin*, p. 16.

20. Anthony Synnott, "Puzzling over the Senses: From Plato to Marx," in David Howes (ed.), *The Varieties of Sensory Experience: A Sourcebook in the Anthropology of the Senses* (Toronto: University of Toronto Press, 1991), p. 63.

21. Synnott, "Puzzling over the Senses," pp. 63–64. While ancient Greek medicine certainly relied on smell, touch, sound, and taste in diagnosing illness, Galenic and later teachings stressed the primacy of the eye, supposedly a thoroughly modern, post-Enlightenment idea. Premodern physicians diagnosed frequently with the eye, at a distance, using written descriptions of symptoms and illustrations. Treatments, too, could be administered from a distance, through written instruction. See, Vivian Nutton, "Galen at the Bedside: The Methods of a Medical Detective," in W. F. Bynum and Roy Porter (eds), *Medicine and the Five Senses* (Cambridge: Cambridge University Press, 1993), pp. 8–9; David Howes, "The Senses in Medicine," *Culture, Medicine and Psychiatry* 19 (1995), p. 127.

22. Synnott, "Puzzling over the Senses," pp. 65–67, 68 (quotation), 69. Medieval Jewish mysticism was, according to Elliot R. Wolfson at least, also much more visual and iconic than is often believed. Wolfson, *Through a Speculum That Shines*.

23. Jane Geaney, *On the Epistemology of the Senses in Early Chinese Thought* (Honolulu: University of Hawai'i Press, 2002), pp. 17, 50–54.

24. Geaney, *On the Epistemology of the Senses in Early Chinese Thought*, pp. 57, 63.

25. Constance Classen, "Sweet Colors, Fragrant Songs: Sensory Models of the Andes and the Amazon," *American Ethnologist* 17 (November 1990), pp. 725, 726.

26. Stephen Houston and Karl Taube, "An Archaeology of the Senses: Perception and Cultural Expression in Ancient Mesoamerica," *Cambridge Archaeological Journal* 10 (2000), pp. 261, 264, 265, 270, 281.

27. Jessica Riskin, *Science in the Age of Sensibility: The Sentimental Empiricists of the French Enlightenment* (Chicago: University of Chicago Press, 2002), pp. 22–23, quotations on 10, 14–15, 61, 65; Roy Porter, *Flesh in the Age of Reason: The Modern Foundations of Body and Soul* (New York: W. W. Norton, 2003), pp. 25–26; Synnott, "Puzzling over the Senses," p. 70; Pallasmaa, *The Eyes of the Skin*, p. 10.

28. Classen, "The Senses," p. 360; Classen, *The Color of Angels*, pp. 98–106. See, too, Irigaray, *Speculum of the other Woman*.

29. Martin Kemp, "'The Mark of Truth': Looking and Learning in some Anatomical Illustrations from the Renaissance and Eighteenth Century," in W. F. Bynum and Roy Porter (eds), *Medicine and the Five Senses* (Cambridge: Cambridge University Press, 1993); Ludmilla Jordanova, "The Art and Science of Seeing in Medicine: Physiognomy 1780–1820," in W. F. Bynum and Roy Porter (eds), *Medicine and the Five Senses*; Malcolm Nicolson, "The Introduction of Percussion and Stethoscopy to Early Nineteenth-Century Edinburgh," in W. F. Bynum and Roy Porter (eds), *Medicine and the Five Senses*; Susan C. Lawrence, "Educating the Senses: Students, Teachers and Medical Rhetoric in Eighteenth-Century London," in W. F. Bynum and Roy Porter (eds), *Medicine and the Five Senses*; Roy Porter, "The Rise of Physical Examination," in W. F. Bynum and Roy Porter (eds), *Medicine and the Five Senses*; Stanley J. Reiser, "Technology and the Use of the Senses in Twentieth-Century Medicine," in W. F. Bynum and Roy Porter (eds), *Medicine and the Five Senses*; Richard Palmer, "In Bad Odor: Smell and its Significance in Medicine from Antiquity to the Seventeenth Century," in W. F. Bynum and Roy Porter (eds), *Medicine and the Five Senses*; Howes, "The Senses in Medicine," p. 132.

30. D. R. Woolf, "Speech, Text, and Time: The Sense of Hearing and the Sense of the Past in Renaissance England" *Albion* 18 (1986), pp. 159–160, 193. Note, too, Goody, *The Interface between the Written and the Oral*; Elizabeth Eisenstein, *The Printing Press as an Agent of Change: Communications and Cultural transformations in Early Modern Europe* (Cambridge: Cambridge University Press, 1979).

31. Flint, *The Victorians and the Visual Imagination*, pp. 2, 3, 8–9, 23, 30–33, quotation on 5. Jonathan Crary offers a similar though more radical argument, pointing out that doubts about the eye and objectivity emerged in the early nineteenth century. See his *Techniques of the Observer*, pp. 3–8, 40–60. Also of relevance here is Gillian Beer, "'Authentic Tidings of Invisible Things': Vision and the Invisible in the Later Nineteenth Century," in Teresa Brennan and Martin Jay (eds), *Vision in Context: Historical and Contemporary Perspectives on Sight* (New York: Routledge, 1996); Brownlee, Peter, "The Economy of the Eyes: Vision and the Cultural Production of Market Revolution, 1800–1860," Ph.D. dissertation, George Washington University, 2003, pp. 12–15 esp.; and, generally, James W. Cook, *The Arts of Deception: Playing with Fraud in the Age of Barnum* (Cambridge, MA: Harvard University Press, 2001).

32. Flint, *The Victorians and the Visual Imagination*, pp. 1, 7, 13, 15, 18. On others sources of the doubt, particularly in European and American philosophy, see Jay, *Downcast Eyes*, p. 14, n.41.

33. Flint, *The Victorians and the Visual Imagination*, pp. 34, 134, 157, 159, 165.

34. Nead, Lynda, *Victorian Babylon: People, Streets and Images in Nineteenth-Century London* (New Haven, CT: Yale University Press, 2000).

35. Flint, *The Victorians and the Visual Imagination*, p. 26; John M. Picker, *Victorian Soundscapes* (New York: Oxford University Press, 2003), pp. 6–14; Jay, *Downcast Eyes*, pp. 3–4.

36. Mark M. Smith, *How Race Is Made*, pp. 166–167 n.12. See also Shawn Michelle Smith, *American Archives: Gender, Race, and Class in Visual Culture* (Princeton, NJ: Princeton University Press, 1999); Shawn Michelle Smith, *Photography on the Color Line: W. E. B. Du Bois, Race, and Visual Culture* (Durham, NC: Duke University Press, 2004); Martin A. Berger, *Sight Unseen: Whiteness and American Visual Culture* (Berkeley: University of California Press, 2005).

37. Smith, *How Race Is Made*, pp. 73–74.

38. Smith, *How Race Is Made*, p. 75.

39. In this particular context, the so-called "lower" senses operated in an emotionally meaningful and powerful fashion, the context itself, the historical associations, and the imperatives of southern segregated society helping to invest ideas about, for example, smell and race with visceral, emotional meaning. I do not mean to suggest that the non-visual senses were inherently "emotional." As a good deal of this book shows, the meaning of the senses was context-driven and the putatively "lower" senses often held intellectual meaning, depending on the particular historical context. Conversely, sight – supposedly the supremely rational sense – could assume visceral meaning, again depending on context. See Angela Rosenthal, "*Visceral* Culture: Blushing and the Legibility of Whiteness in Eighteenth-Century British Portraiture," in Deborah Curry (ed.), *Art: History: Visual: Culture* (Malden, MA: Blackwell, 2005), pp. 85–112.

40. Andrei Toporkov, "The Devil's Candle? Street Lighting," *History Today* 46 (November 1996), p. 36. See, also, Carolyn Korsmeyer, *Making Sense of Taste: Food and Philosophy* (Ithaca, NY: Cornell University Press, 1999).

41. Samuel Martland, "Progress Illuminating the World: Street Lighting in Santiago, Valparaiso and La Plata, 1840–1890," *Urban History* 29 (2002), quotations on p. 223.

Chapter 2 Hearing

1. See, especially, Michael Bull and Les Back (eds), *The Auditory Culture Reader* (Oxford: Berg, 2003); Viet Erlmann (ed.), *Hearing Cultures: Essays on Sound, Listening and Modernity* (Oxford: Berg, 2004); Jim Drobnick (ed.), *Aural Cultures* (Toronto: YYZ Books, 2004). I elaborate on some of the issues addressed in this

chapter in my "Introduction: Onward to Audible Pasts," in Mark M. Smith (ed.), *Hearing History: A Reader* (Athens, GA: University of Georgia Press, 2004).

2. Attali, Jacques, *Noise: The Political Economy of Music*, Brian Maussumi (trans.) (Minneapolis: University of Minnesota Press, 1985), pp. 3–20 esp.

3. Douglas Kahn, "Art and Sound," in Mark M. Smith (ed.), *Hearing History: A Reader* (Athens, GA: University of Georgia Press, 2004), pp. 36–37. Even more surprising, perhaps, are continuing calls for more historical studies of music even as historians have made the sensible and entirely needed shift to a broader, more expansive definition of sound that includes, but is not defined by, music. For a call by an American historian for a return to the study of music, see Scott Gac, "Listening to the Progressives," *Reviews in American History* 32 (September 2004), pp. 410–411.

4. Hibbitts, "Coming to Our Senses," [2.14–2.15], [2.24].

5. Hibbitts, "Coming to Our Senses," [2.6, 2.3]; Rath, *How Early America Sounded*, pp. 51–52, 56–57.

6. Synnott, "Puzzling over the Senses," p. 67; Classen, "The Senses," p. 359; Nutton, "Galen at the Bedside," p. 11; Liz James, "Senses and Sensibility in Byzantium," in *Art: History: Visual: Culture*, Deborah Curry (ed.) (Malden, MA: Blackwell, 2005), p. 49.

7. Hibbitts, "Coming to Our Senses," [2.17, 2.18].

8. Charles Burnett, "Perceiving Sound in the Middle Ages," in Mark M. Smith (ed.), *Hearing History: A Reader* (Athens, GA: University of Georgia Press, 2004), pp. 69–84.

9. Penelope Gouk, "Some English Theories of Hearing in the Seventeenth Century: Before and After Descartes," in Charles Burnett, Michael Fend, and Penelope Gouk (eds), *The Second Sense: Studies in Hearing and Musical Judgement from Antiquity to the Seventeenth Century* (London: Warburg Institute, 1991), pp. 95–113

10. David Garrioch, "Sounds of the City: The Soundscape of Early Modern European Towns," *Urban History* 30 (2003), esp. p. 11; Jacques Le Goff, "Merchant's Time and Church's Time in the Middle Ages," in Jacques Le Goff, *Time, Work, and Culture in the Middle Ages* (Chicago: University of Chicago Press, 1980); Gerhard Dohrn-van Rossum, *History of the Hour: Clocks and Modern Temporal Orders* (Chicago: University of Chicago Press, 1996); David S., Landes, *Revolution in Time: Clocks and the Making of the Modern World* (Cambridge, MA: Harvard University Press, 1983).

11. Bruce R. Smith, *The Acoustic World of Early Modern England: Attending to the O-Factor* (Chicago: University Press of Chicago, 1999), pp. 49–95.

12. Rath, *How Early America Sounded*, pp. 104–106.

13. C. Mackenzie Brown, "Purāna as Scripture: From Sound to Image of the Holy Word in the Hindu Tradition," *History of Religions* 26 (August 1986); Classen, "Sweet Colors, Fragrant Songs," pp. 723, 724.

14. Ruth Finnegan, *Communicating: The Multiple Modes of Human Interconnection* (London: Routledge, 2002), pp. 72–73; Philip D. Morgan, *Slave Counterpoint:*

Black Culture in the Eighteenth-Century Chesapeake and Lowcountry (Chapel Hill: University of North Carolina Press, 1998), pp. 418–420, 581, 594.

15. George Devereux, "Ethnopsychological Aspects of the Terms 'Deaf' and 'Dumb'," in David Howes (ed.) *Sensual Relations: Engaging the Senses in Culture and Social Theory* (Ann Arbor: University of Michigan Press, 2003), quotations, in order, pp. 43, 44, 45.

16. Steven Feld, *Sound and Sentiment: Birds, Weeping, Poetics and Song in Kaluli Expression* (Philadelphia: University of Pennsylvania Press, 1990). See, also, Paul Stoller, "Sound in Songhay Cultural Experience," *American Ethnologist* 11 (1984).

17. Daniel, "The Pulse as an Icon in Siddha Medicine," p. 108; Nicolson, "The Introduction of Percussion and Stethoscopy to Early Nineteenth-Century Edinburgh," pp. 134–153.

18. Alain Corbin, *Village Bells: Sound and Meaning in the 19th-Century French Countryside*, Martin Thom (trans.) (New York: Columbia University Press, 1998), pp. xv–xvii, 80–93, 110–118, 391–392, 306–307, quotations on pp. 3, 299; E. P. Thompson, "Rough Music," in his *Customs in Common* (London: Merlin Press, 1991), pp. 467–538.

19. Mark M. Smith, *Listening to Nineteenth-Century America* (Chapel Hill: University of North Carolina Press, 2001), pp. 93–260.

20. Nicholas Vazsonyi, "Hegemony Through Harmony: German Identity, Music, and Enlightenment around 1800," in Nora M. Alter and Lutz Koepnick (eds), *Sound Matters: Essays on the Acoustics of Modern German Culture* (Oxford: Berghahn Books, 2004), pp. 35–36; Nora M. Alter, and Lutz Koepnick, "Introduction: Sound Matters," in Nora M. Alter and Lutz Koepnick (eds), *Sound Matters: Essays on the Acoustics of Modern German Culture* (Oxford: Berghahn Books, 2004), pp. 10, 11.

21. Parr, "Notes for a More Sensuous History," p. 740.

22. James H. Johnson, *Listening in Paris: A Cultural History*, Studies on the History of Society and Culture, 21 (Berkeley: University of California Press, 1995), pp. 3, 81 (quotations), 82–95, 228–236.

23. Smith, *Listening to Nineteenth-Century America*, pp. 19–46.

24. Shane White and Graham White, "'I was nearly stunned by the noise he made': Listening to African American Religious Sound in the Era of Slavery," *American Nineteenth Century History*, 1 (Spring 2000), pp. 34–61; David W. Blight, "'Analyze the Sounds': Frederick Douglass' Invitation to Modern Historians of Slavery," in Stephan Palmié (ed.), *Slave Cultures and the Cultures of Slavery* (Knoxville: University of Tennessee Press, 1995); Jon Cruz, *Culture on the Margins: The Black Spiritual and the Rise of American Cultural Interpretation* (Princeton, NJ: Princeton University Press, 1999).

25. Smith, *Listening to Nineteenth Century America*, pp. 66–91.

26. Leigh Eric Schmidt, *Hearing Things: Religion, Illusions, and the American Enlightenment* (Cambridge, MA: Harvard University Press, 2000), pp. 66 (quotation), 38–77 esp.

27. Schmidt, *Hearing Things*, pp. 39–45.

28. Raymond Smilor, "Confronting the Industrial Environment: The Noise Problem in America, 1893–1932." Ph.D. dissertation, University of Texas, 1978, pp. 3–38; Raymond Smilor, "Personal Boundaries in the Urban Environment: The Legal Attack on Noise: 1865–1930," *Environmental Review*, 3 (1979), pp. 24–36; Raymond Smilor, "Toward an Environmental Perspective: The Anti-Noise Campaign, 1883–1932," in Martin V. Melosi (ed.), *Pollution and Reform in American Cities, 1870–1930* (Austin: University of Texas Press, 1980), pp. 135–151.

29. Smilor, "Personal Boundaries in the Urban Environment," pp. 24–36.

30. On the English case, John M. Picker, "The Soundproof Study: Victorian Professionals, Work Space, and Urban Noise," *Victorian Studies* 42 (Spring 1999/2000); Jon Agar, "Bodies, Machines and Noise," in Iwan Rhys Morus (ed.) *Bodies/Machines* (Oxford: Berg, 2002). On Germany, Lawrence Baron, "Noise and Degeneration: Theodor Lessing's Crusade for Quiet," *Journal of Contemporary History* 17 (January 1982).

31. Emily Thompson, *The Soundscape of Modernity: Architectural Acoustics and the Culture of Listening in America, 1900–1933* (Cambridge, MA: MIT Press, 2002), pp. 170, 171.

32. Thompson, *Soundscape of Modernity*, pp. 2, 4, 171–172.

33. Jonathan Sterne, *The Audible Past: Cultural Origins of Sound Reproduction* (Durham, NC: Duke University Press, 2003), pp. 287–408.

34. Lisa Gitelman, *Scripts, Grooves, and Writing Machines: Representing Technology in the Edison Era* (Stanford, CA: Stanford University Press, 1999), pp. 119–147; Sterne, *The Audible Past*, pp. 402–208; Smith, *How Race Is Made*, ch.5; Paul Gilroy, *Against Race: Imagining Political Culture Beyond the Color Line* (Cambridge: Belknap Press of Harvard University Press, 2000). For work on the post-1945 period, see especially, Douglas Kahn, *Noise, Water, Meat: A History of Sound in the Arts* (Cambridge, MA: MIT Press, 1999).

35. Keletso E. Atkins, *The Moon Is Dead! Give Us Our Money! The Cultural Origins of an African Work Ethic, Natal, South Africa, 1843–1900* (Portsmouth, NH: Heinemann, 1993), pp. 86–96; Mark M. Smith, "Old South Time in Comparative Perspective," *American Historical Review* 101 (December 1996); Sandra Lauderdale Graham, *House and Street: The Domestic World of Servants and Masters in Nineteenth-Century Rio de Janeiro* (Austin: University of Texas Press, 1992).

36. Graeme Davison, *The Unforgiving Minute: How Australia Learned to Tell the Time* (New York: Oxford University Press, 1993), pp. 24–28; Paul Carter, *The Sound In-Between: Voice, Space, Performance* (New South Wales: New South Wales University Press and New Endeavour Press, 1992), quotations, in order, pp. 21, 27, 28, 29. See also Joy Damousi, "'The Filthy American Twang': Elocution, the Advent of American 'Talkies,' and Australian Cultural Identity," *American Historical Review* 112 (April 2007), pp. 394–416.

Chapter 3 Smelling

1. Constance Classen, Howes, David, and Synnott, Anthony, *Aroma: The Cultural History of Smell* (New York: Routledge, 1994), pp. ii (quotation), 3, 7, 8. The recent collection Jim Drobnick (ed.), *The Smell Culture Reader* (Oxford: Berg, 2006) suggests that the topic is beginning to attract scholarly interest.

2. Classen, *Worlds of Sense*, pp. 30–31, 7; Anthony Synnott, "A Sociology of Smell," *Canadian Review of Sociology and Anthropology* 28 (November 1991); Stephen Kern, "Olfactory Ontology and Scented Harmonies: On the History of Smell," *Journal of Popular Culture* 4 (Spring 1974), p. 819; Jay Geller, "'A glance at the nose': Freud's Inscription of Jewish Difference," *American Imago* 49, no.4.

3. Ian D. Ritchie, "The Nose Knows: Bodily Knowing in Isaiah 11.3," *Journal for the Study of the Old Testament* 87 (2000), p. 73; Classen, *Worlds of Sense*, pp. 17–18.

4. Classen, "The Senses," p. 360; Nutton, "Galen at the Bedside," p. 8.

5. Béatrice Caseau, "The Use and Meaning of Fragrance in the Ancient World and their Christianization (100–900 AD)," Ph.D dissertation, Princeton University, 1994, pp. iv, 3–2, 33–36.

6. Ritchie, "The Nose Knows," p. 59, quotation on p. 61; Classen, *Worlds of Sense*, pp. 19, 21.

7. Caseau, "The Use and Meaning of Fragrances in the Ancient World," pp. 1–3, quotations on p. 4; Susan Ashbrook Harvey, *Scenting Salvation: Ancient Christianity and the Olfactory Imagination* (Berkeley: University of California Press, 2006), pp. 25–26.

8. Susan Ashbrook Harvey, "St. Ephrem on the Scent of Salvation," *Journal of Theological Studies* 49 (April 1998), quotation on p. 113; Susan Ashbrook Harvey, *Scenting Salvation*, pp. 60–64, 182, 235–239.

9. Classen, *Worlds of Sense*, pp. 19 (quotation), 20.

10. Classen, *Worlds of Sense*, pp. 7–8; Peter Gay, *The Bourgeois Experience. Victoria to Freud. Volume 1. Education of the Senses* (New York: Oxford University Press, 1984), p. 415.

11. Classen, *Worlds of Sense*, pp. 22–23, 28.

12. Jeffrey Chipps Smith, *Sensuous Worship: Jesuits and the Art of the Early Catholic Reformation in Germany* (Princeton, NJ: Princeton University Press, 2002), pp. 1, 3, 29, 35 (first two quotations), 39 (last quotation), 40; David Howes, "Olfaction and Transition," in David Howes (ed.), *The Varieties of Sensory Experience: A Sourcebook in the Anthropology of the Senses* (Toronto: University of Toronto Press), 1991, p. 129; Classen, "The Senses," pp. 359, 360; Classen, *Worlds of Sense*, p. 17.

13. Mark S. R. Jenner, "Civilization and Deodorization? Smell in Early Modern English Culture," in Peter Burke, Brian Harrison, and Paul Slack (eds), *Civil Histories: Essays Presented to Sir Keith Thomas* (New York: Oxford University Press, 2000), pp. 131 (quotation), 132–133, 136.

14. Classen, *Worlds of Sense*, pp. 28 (quotation), 9–10, 87–88, 31; Brenda Farnell, "Kinesthetic Sense and Dynamically Embodied Action," *Journal for the Anthropological Study of Human Movement*," 12 (2003), p. 133.

15. Classen, *Worlds of Sense*, pp. 81–83, quotation on p. 82.

16. Howes, "Olfaction and Transition," p. 145.

17. Corbin, *The Foul and the Fragrant*, pp. 77–85, 94–96, 140–141, 199, 231–232; David Howes, "Scent and Sensibility," *Culture, Medicine and Psychiatry* 13 (1989), p. 93; Sima Godfrey, "Alain Corbin: Making Sense of French History," *French Historical Studies* 25 (Spring 2002), p. 385; David S. Barnes, *The Great Stink of Paris and the Nineteenth-Century Struggle against Filth and Disease* (Baltimore, MD: The Johns Hopkins University Press, 2006).

18. Corbin, *Time, Desire, Horror*, 147; David Garrioch, *The Making of Revolutionary France* (Berkeley: University of California Press, 2004), pp. 16–18, 214–216; Jenner, "Civilization and Deodorization?" p. 137.

19. Corbin, *Time, Desire, Horror*, pp. 153, 165; Barnes, *The Great Stink of Paris and the Nineteenth-Century Struggle against Filth and Disease*.

20. Corbin, *Time, Desire, Horror*, p. 155.

21. Christine Meisner Rosen, "'Knowing' Industrial Pollution: Nuisance Law and the Power of Tradition in a Time of Rapid Economic Change, 1840–1864," *Environmental History* 8 (October 2003), pp. 568–569, 571 (quotation), 574–575, 577, 587–588.

22. Martland, "Constructing Valparaiso," pp. 138–141, quotation on p. 139.

23. See Gale Peter Largey and David Rodney Watson, "The Sociology of Odors," *American Journal of Sociology* 77 (May 1972), p. 1026.

24. Connie Y. Chiang, "Monterey-by-the-Smell: Odors and Social Conflict on the California Coastline," *Pacific Historical Review* 73 (May 2004), quotations, in order, pp. 192, 185.

25. Chiang, "Monterey-by-the-Smell," pp. 203–210, quotation on p. 214.

26. Graham, *House and Street*, quotations on pp. 116–117, 118–119.

27. J. C. Peters, *The Science & Art, or the Principles & Practice of Medicine* (New York: William Raddle, n.d.), vol. 1, p. 4.

28. Mark M. Smith, *How Race Is Made*, pp. 66–78.

29. Mark M. Smith, *How Race Is Made*, pp. 98–113; Classen, "The Senses," p. 356.

30. Timothy Burke, *Lifebuoy Men, Lux Women: Commodification, Consumption, and Cleanliness in Modern Zimbabwe* (Durham, NC: Duke University Press, 1996), pp. 20–24, 37.

31. Matthew J. Payne, *Stalin's Railroad: Turksib and the Building of Socialism* (Pittsburgh: University of Pittsburgh Press, 2001), p. 146.

32. Classen, *Worlds of Sense*, pp. 31, 92; Informant 9F, "Russian Sensory Images," pp. 164–165, 166. On American olfactory blandness, see Edward T. Hall, *The Hidden Dimension* (New York: Doubleday, 1969), pp. 45–46. On immigrants and olfactory stereotypes in Britain after the Second World War, see Largey and Watson, "The Sociology of Odors," p. 1023.

Chapter 4 Tasting

1. Sidney W. Mintz, "Time, Sugar, and Sweetness," *Marxist Perspectives* 2 (Winter 1979/80), p. 56; Barbara Fischer, "Introduction," in Barbara Fischer (ed.), *Tasting Identities and Geographies in Art* (Toronto: YYZ Books, 1999), p. 21; Sidney W. Mintz, *Sweetness and Power: The Place of Sugar in Modern History* (New York: Viking, 1987); Wolfgang Schivelbusch, *Tastes of Paradise: A Social History of Spices, Stimulants, and Intoxicants*, David Jacobson (trans.) (New York: Vintage Books, 1992); Peter Macinnis, *Bittersweet: The Story of Sugar*, (St. Leonards, NSW: Allen & Unwin, 2002); Mark Kurlansky, *Salt: A World History* (New York: Penguin, 2002); Andrew Dalby, *Dangerous Tastes: The Story of Spices* (Berkeley: University of California Press, 2000); Sidney W. Mintz, *Tasting Food, Tasting Freedom: Excursions into Eating, Culture, and the Past* (Boston: Beacon Press, 1996). For key work by students of philosophy and literature, see Korsmeyer, *Making Sense of Taste*; Denise Gigante, *Taste: A Literary History* (New Haven, CT: Yale University Press, 2005). Quotation from Korsmeyer, "Introduction: Perspectives on Tastes," in Carolyn Korsmeyer (ed.), *The Taste Culture Reader: Experiencing Food and Drink* (Oxford: Berg, 2005), p. 4.

2. Hibbitts, "Coming to Our Senses," [2.67, 2.69, 2.71]; Nutton, "Galen at the Bedside," p. 11.

3. Korsmeyer, *Making Sense of Taste*, pp. 5, 16–17, 22–23, 30–33; Korsmeyer, "Introduction: Perspectives on Tastes," p. 2; T. Sarah Peterson, *Acquired Taste: The French Origins of Modern Cooking* (Ithaca, NY: Cornell University Press, 1994), p. 47.

4. J.-P. Vernant "Introduction," in Marcel Detienne, *The Gardens of Adonis: Spices in Greek Mythology*, Janet Lloyd (trans.) (Princeton, NJ: Princeton University Press, 1994), p. xi, quotation on p. xii; Marcel Detienne, *The Gardens of Adonis*.

5. Jack Goody, "The High and the Low: Culinary Culture in Asia and Europe," Carolyn Korsmeyer (ed.) in *The Taste Culture Reader: Experiencing Food and Drink* (Oxford: Berg, 2005), p. 58, quotations on p. 60.

6. Alan Hunt, *Governance of the Consuming Passions: A History of Sumptuary Law* (New York: St. Martin's Press, 1996), pp. 1, 8; Goody, "The High and the Low: Culinary Culture in Asia and Europe," pp. 67, 68.

7. Synnott, "Puzzling over the Senses," pp. 67, 69; Boyd Taylor Coolman, *Knowing God by Experience: The Spiritual Senses in the Theology of William of Auxerre* (Washington, DC: Catholic University of America Press, 2004), p. 219.

8. Goody, "The High and the Low: Culinary Culture in Asia and Europe," pp. 58–59.

9. Peterson, *Acquired Taste*, pp. 2–3, quotations on pp. 11–12, 14; Schivelbusch, *Tastes of Paradise*, pp. 4–5.

10. Peterson, *Acquired Taste*, pp. 45–46, 51, quotations on pp. 49–50.

11. Peterson, *Acquired Taste*, pp. 187, 183, 193, 198.

12. Jennifer Fisher, "Performing Taste," in Barbara Fischer (ed.), *Tasting Identities and Geographies in Art* (Toronto: YYZ Books, 1999), quotations, in order, on pp. 29, 31, 32.

13. David Howes and Marc Lalonde, "The History of Sensibilities: Of the Standard of Taste In Mid-Eighteenth Century England and the Circulation of Smells in Post-Revolutionary France," *Dialectical Anthropology* 16 (1991), p. 125.

14. Howes and Lalonde, "The History of Sensibilities," pp. 126–128.

15. Howes and Lalonde, "The History of Sensibilities," pp. 128–130, first quotation on p. 129, second and third on p. 130; Mark M. Smith, *How Race Is Made*, ch.5.

16. Mintz, "Time, Sugar, and Sweetness," p. 57.

17. Mintz, "Time, Sugar, and Sweetness," pp. 58–59, quotation on p. 58.

18. Mintz, "Time, Sugar, and Sweetness," quotations on pp. 59, 60.

19. Donna R. Gabbacia, "Colonial Creoles: The Formation of Tastes in Early America," in Carolyn Korsmeyer (ed.), *The Taste Culture Reader: Experiencing Food and Drink* (Oxford: Berg, 2005), pp. 79, 80–81.

20. Gabaccia, "Colonial Creoles," pp. 81, 82, 83.

21. Gabaccia, "Colonial Creoles," pp. 84, 85.

22. James E. McWilliams, *A Revolution in Eating: How the Quest for Food Shaped America* (New York: Columbia University Press, 2005), pp. 8 (quotation), 9.

23. McWilliams, *Revolution in Eating*, p. 83.

24. McWilliams, *Revolution in Eating*, pp. 304–308, 313, quotations on pp. 309, 311.

25. David Sutton, "Listen to that Scent! Travelling Tastes and Smells Among Greek Immigrants," *Detours Online Magazine*, 5 (May 2003). See also his "Sensory Memory and the Construction of 'Worlds'," in *Remembrance of Repasts: An Anthropology of Food and Memory* (Oxford: Berg, 2001), pp. 73–102.

26. Karl Gerth, "Commodifying Chinese Nationalism: MSG and the Flavor of Patriotic Production," in Susan Strasser (ed.), *Commodifying Everything: Relationships of the Market* (New York: Routledge, 2003), pp. 235–238, quotation on p. 235.

27. Gerth, "Commodifying Chinese Nationalism," pp. 243, 246–247.

28. Mark S. Swislocki, "Feast and Famine in Republican Shanghai: Urban Food Culture, Nutrition, and the State," Ph.D. dissertation, Stanford University, 2002, pp. 3–5, 55–57.

29. Swislocki, "Feast and Famine in Republican Shanghai," p. 63.

30. Swislocki, "Feast and Famine in Republican Shanghai," pp. 14–18, 21–22. Debates about who got to eat what and how much became an increasingly political and pressing issue later in China, especially at the height of the national famine of 1959–1961, see Judith Farquar, *Appetites: Food and Sex in Post-Socialist China* (Durham, NC: Duke University Press, 2002), pp. 82–83, 122, 130–132.

31. Corbin, *Time, Desire, Horror*, p. 2; Pierre Bourdieu, "Taste of Luxury, Taste of Necessity," in Carolyn Korsmeyer (ed.), *The Taste Culture Reader: Experiencing*

Food and Drink (Oxford: Berg, 2005); Payne, *Stalin's Railroad*, p. 146. For the larger Soviet context and the shaping of a national taste, see Jukka Gronow, "Champagne and Caviar: Soviet Kitsch," in Carolyn Korsmeyer (ed.), *The Taste Culture Reader: Experiencing Food and Drink* (Oxford: Berg, 2005).

32. Joy Parr, "Local Water Diversely Known: Walkerton Ontario, 2000 and After," *Environment and Planning D: Society and Space* 22 (2004), pp. 347–348.

Chapter 5 Touch

1. Hibbitts, "Coming to Our Senses," [2.46]; Constance Classen, "Fingerprints: Writing about Touch," in Constance Classen (ed.), *The Book of Touch* (Oxford: Berg, 2005), pp. 4–6, 7, 13, quotation on p. 5.

2. Geraldine A. Johnson, "Touch, Tactility, and the Reception of Sculpture in Early Modern Italy," in Paul Smith and Carolyn Wilde (eds), *A Companion to Art Theory* (Malden, MA: Blackwell, 2002), pp. 62–63; James Hall, *The World as Sculpture: The Changing Status of Sculpture from the Renaissance to the Present* (London: Chatto and Windus, 1999), pp, 82–103; Anthony Synnott, *The Body Social: Symbolism, Self and Society* (London: Routledge, 1993), pp. 130–150; Elizabeth D. Harvey, "Introduction: The 'Sense of All Senses," in Elizabeth D. Harvey (ed.), *Sensible Flesh: On Touch in Early Modern Culture* (Philadelphia: University of Pennsylvania Press, 2003), pp. 1–2, 15.

3. Parr, "Notes for a More Sensuous History," p. 742; Sander Gilman, "Touch, Sexuality and Disease," in W. F. Bynum and Roy Porter (eds), *Medicine and the Five Senses* (Cambridge: Cambridge University Press, 1993); Sander Gilman, *Goethe's Touch: Touching, Sexuality, and Seeing* (New Orleans: Graduate School of Tulane University, 1988); Marjorie O'Rourke Boyle, *Senses of Touch: Human Dignity and Deformity from Michelangelo to Calvin* (Leiden: Brill, 1998); Laura Gowing, *Common Bodies: Women, Touch and Power in Seventeenth-Century England* (New Haven, CT: Yale University Press, 2003); Elizabeth D. Harvey, (ed.), *Sensible Flesh: On Touch in Early Modern Culture* (Philadelphia: University of Pennsylvania Press, 2003). For literary and theoretical treatments see, most obviously, Steven Connor, *The Book of Skin* (Ithaca, NY: Cornell University Press, 2004); Santanu Das, *Touch and Intimacy in First World War Literature* (New York: Cambridge University Press, 2005).

4. Gilman, "Touch, Sexuality and Disease," pp. 199–200. Note, too Don Ihde, *Sense and Significance* (Pittsburgh: Duquesne University Press, 1973), pp. 97–98.

5. Gilman, "Touch, Sexuality and Disease," p. 199. For some sensible reservations about tethering touch too closely to sight, see Howes, "The Senses in Medicine," p. 131.

6. Gilman, "Touch, Sexuality and Disease," p. 198.

7. Classen, "Fingerprints," pp. 2, 3, first quotation on p. 3; David Chidester, "The American Touch: Tactile Imagery in American Religion and Politics," in Constance Classen (ed.), *The Book of Touch* (Oxford: Berg, 2005), p. 61.

8. Classen, "Fingerprints," p. 7; Brian E. McKnight, "Sung Justice: Death by Slicing," *Journal of the American Oriental Society* 93 (July–September 1973), pp. 359–360.

9. Hibbitts, "Coming to Our Senses," [2.34, 2.54–2.56, 2.58].

10. Nutton, "Galen at the Bedside," p. 11; Classen, "The Senses," p. 360; Daniel, "The Pulse as an Icon in Siddha Medicine," pp. 100–101, 107–108.

11. Gilman, "Touch, Sexuality and Disease," p. 198; Ruth Finnegan, "Tactile Communication," in Constance Classen (ed.), *The Book of Touch* (Oxford: Berg, 2005), p. 19; Hibbitts, "Coming to Our Senses," [2.50].

12. Boyle, *Senses of Touch*, pp. 19–20, 24.

13. Synnott, "Puzzling over the Senses," pp. 68, 69.

14. Gordon Rudy, *Mystical Language of Sensation in the Later Middle Ages* (New York: Routledge, 2002), p. 2. Note, too, Louise Vinge, *The Five Senses: Studies in a Literary Tradition* (Lund: CWK Gleerup, 1975), pp. 26–27.

15. Rudy, *Mystical Language*, pp. 4, 5, 8–9. Rudy's is a thoughtful book although historiographically quirky. He picks unnecessary fights with others working on the senses and fails to explain precisely why he finds their work unhelpful. See, for example, pp. 9, 127 note 4.

16. Rudy, *Mystical Language*, pp. 56–57 (first quotation), 58, 59, 61 (second quotation); Coolman, *Knowing God by Experience*, pp. 139–141.

17. Gilman, "Touch, Sexuality and Disease," pp. 202, 209, 210, 215–216; Gilman, *Goethe's Touch*, p. 3.

18. Gilman, *Goethe's Touch*, pp. 8, 9.

19. Eve Keller, "The Subject of Touch: Medical Authority in Early Modern Midwifery," in Elizabeth D. Harvey (ed.), *Sensible Flesh: On Touch in Early Modern Culture* (Philadelphia: University of Pennsylvania Press, 2003), pp. 62–63, 69, 71, 80; Porter, "The Rise of Physical Examination," p. 179.

20. Laura Gowing, *Common Bodies: Women, Touch and Power in Seventeenth-Century England* (New Haven, CT: Yale University Press, 2003), quotation on p. 6.

21. Gowing, *Common Touch*, pp. 53–56, 149–173.

22. Elliot J. Gorn, "'Gouge and bite, pull hair and scratch': The Social Significance of Fighting in the Southern Backcountry," *American Historical Review* 90 (1985). On the British, see Ridley and Goodchild, "Bare-knuckle is all the rage," *Independent on Sunday*, September 19, 1999, p. 3.

23. Norbert Elias, *The History of Manners*, vol.1: *The Civilizing Process*, Edmund Jephcott (trans.) (New York, 1982); Elizabeth D. Harvey, "Introduction: The Sense of All Senses," p. 9.

24. Gilman, *Goethe's Touch*, p. 4.

25. John E. Crowley, *The Invention of Comfort: Sensibilities and Design in Early Modern Britain and Early America* (Baltimore, MD: Johns Hopkins University Press, 2001), quotation on p. 142.

26. Crowley, *The Invention of Comfort*, pp. 142–143, 166–168.

27. Crowley, *The Invention of Comfort*, pp. 146–150, 162–165, quotations on p. 157.

28. Elizabeth D. Harvey, "Introduction: The Sense of All Senses," p. 10; Finnegan, "Tactile Communication," p. 22; Keith Thomas, "Magical Healing: The King's Touch," in Constance Classen (ed.), *The Book of Touch* (Oxford: Berg, 2005), p. 355; Marc Bloch, *The Royal Touch: Monarchy and Miracles in France and England* (New York: Dorset Press, 1989).

29. Thomas, "Magical Healing," p. 355, quotation on pp. 355–356.

30. Finnegan, "Tactile Communication," p. 20–21; Richard Bauman, *Let Your Words Be Few: Symbolism of Speaking and Silence Among Seventeenth-Century Quakers* (Cambridge: Cambridge University Press, 1983), p. 47. Note, too, Howes, "Skinscapes: Embodiment, Culture, and Environment," in Constance Classen (ed.), *The Book of Touch* (Oxford: Berg, 2005), p. 27.

31. Chidester, "The American Touch," p. 51, quotations on p. 52.

32. Chidester, "The American Touch," p. 53.

33. Mark M. Smith, "The Skin-Man: Getting in Touch with Abraham Lincoln." (Work in progress: in author's possession).

34. Hunt, *Governance of the Consuming Passions*, pp. 23–24.

35. For a wonderful book linking clothing and politics but which suffers from the hyper-visualism of what was worn, see Michael Zakim, *Ready-Made Democracy: A History of Men's Dress in the American Republic, 1760–1860* (Chicago: University of Chicago Press, 2003).

36. Peter Charles Hoffer, *Sensory Worlds of Early America* (Baltimore, MD: Johns Hopkins University Press, 2004), pp. 234–236, 241, quotation on p. 235.

37. Details on fustian, O'Connor, and Engels from Peter Stallybrass, "Marx's Coat," in Patricia Spyer (ed.), *Border Fetishisms: Material Objects in Unstable Places* (New York: Routledge, 1998), pp. 183–207, 192–193 especially.

38. Peter Stallybrass and Allon White, "Bourgeois Perception: The Gaze and the Contaminating Touch," in Constance Classen (ed.), *The Book of Touch* (Oxford: Berg, 2005), pp. 289–291.

39. Corbin, *Time, Desire, Horror*, pp. 191–192, 188.

40. Constance Classen, "Feminine Tactics: Crafting and Alternative Aesthetics in the Eighteenth and Nineteenth Centuries," in Constance Classen (ed.), *The Book of Touch* (Oxford: Berg, 2005), pp. 228–232, quotations on p. 229.

41. Associations between blackness and tactility seem to have been medieval in origin. Also, as Gilman explains, leprosy was believed to turn skin black. "Blackness marks the sufferer from disease, sets him outside the world of purity and cleanliness" and also denotes his inferiority and suggests sexual deviancy and inability to resist the allure of the skin, for which his skin, in turn, pays the "price" of bodily enslavement (Gilman, "Touch, Sexuality and Disease," p. 202). See also Gilroy, *Against Race*.

42. Mark M. Smith, *How Race Is Made*, ch.1.

43. Gilman, "Touch, Sexuality and Disease," pp. 216–223, quotation on p. 224.

44. Scott Manning Stevens, "New World Contacts and the Trope of the 'Naked Savage'," in Elizabeth D. Harvey (ed.), *Sensible Flesh: On Touch in Early Modern*

Culture (Philadelphia: University of Pennsylvania Press, 2003), quotations on 126, 127.

45. Stevens, "New World Contacts," pp. 130–132, 135, quotation on p. 130; Hoffer, *Sensory Worlds*, p. 32.

46. C. E. Tyndale-Biscoe, "The Imperial Touch: Schooling Male Bodies in Colonial India, Part I," in Constance Classen (ed.), *The Book of Touch* (Oxford: Berg, 2005), pp. 168–170, quotation on p. 169; Satadru Sen, "The Imperial Touch: Schooling Male Bodies in Colonial India, Part II," in Constance Classen (ed.), *The Book of Touch*, pp. 171–176.

47. Anthony Synnott, "Handling Children: To Touch or Not to Touch?," in Constance Classen (ed.), *The Book of Touch* (Oxford: Berg, 2005), p. 41.

48. Synnott, "Handling Children," pp. 42–47; Gay, *The Bourgeois Experience*, pp. 437–440; Katherine C. Grier, *Culture and Comfort: Parlor Making and Middle-Class Identity, 1850–1930* (Washington, DC: Smithsonian Institution Press, 1997).

49. Klaus Theweleit, "Sexuality and the Drill: The Body Reconstructed in the Military Academy," in Constance Classen (ed.), *The Book of Touch* (Oxford: Berg, 2005), pp. 178–185.

50. Das, *Touch and Intimacy*.

51. Geraldine A. Johnson, "Touch, Tactility, and the Reception of Sculpture," pp. 64–65, 70–71, quotation on p. 61; Yi-Fu Tuan Tuan, "The Pleasures of Touch," in Constance Classen (ed.), *The Book of Touch* (Oxford: Berg, 2005), p. 77.

52. Pallasmaa, *The Eyes of the Skin*, pp. 24–25; Martin Jay, "Scopic Regimes of Modernity," in Hal Foster (ed.), *Vision and Visuality* (Seattle, WA: Bay Press, 1988), p. 18; Ghiberti quoted in Classen and Howes, "The Museum as Sensescape," n.p. For the sensory extreme in modern art, installations that not only downplay light but up the sensory ante, see Stephen Di Benedetto, "Stumbling in the Dark: Facets of Sensory Perception and Robert Wilson's 'H.G.' Installation," *New Theatre Quarterly* 67 (2001). Note also Jennifer Fisher, "Relational Sense: Towards a Haptic Aesthetics," *Parachute* 87 (Summer 1997).

53. Cohen Bull, "Sense, Meaning, and Perception," p. 275.

54. Classen and Howes, "The Museum as Sensescape," n.p.; Constance Classen, "Museum Manners: The Sensory Life of the Early Museum," *Journal of Social History* 40 (June 2007), 895–914.

55. Fiona Candlin, "Don't Touch! Hands Off! Art, Blindness and the Conservation of Expertise," *Body and Society* 10 (2004), p. 72.

56. Jennifer Price, "Looking for Nature at the Mall: A Field Guide to the Nature Company," in William Cronon (ed.), *Uncommon Ground: Toward Reinventing Nature* (New York: W. W. Norton, 1995), p. 196; Susan G. Davis, "Touch the Magic," in *Uncommon Ground: Toward Reinventing Nature*, William Cronon (ed.) (New York: W. W. Norton, 1995).

Conclusion: Future of Senses Past

1. I have wrestled with these questions in my own work. My first effort to deal with the history of sound in nineteenth-century America, for example, sometimes relied too heavily on psychoacoustics to unravel the contemporary meanings of soundscapes, a methodology that can, without due care, blur the distinction between past and present (see my *Listening to Nineteenth-Century America*, pp. 266–267). My subsequent thinking has moved toward a more constructionist – and historical – treatment of the senses. My most recent thinking – which informs a good deal of this conclusion – is outlined in my essay "Producing Sense, Consuming Sense, Making Sense."

2. Jütte, *History of the Senses*, pp. 8, 9; Classen, "The Senses," p. 357.

3. Jütte, *History of the Senses*, pp. 8, 9.

4. Hoffer, *Sensory Worlds*, pp. 2, 6.

5. Hoffer, *Sensory Worlds*, pp. 2, 8, 9, 10.

6. Hoffer, *Sensory Worlds*, p. 253; Jütte, *History of the Senses*, pp. 1–3.

7. See http://www.history.org/visit/eventsAndExhibits/holidays/christmas.cfm (accessed 11 December 2006).

8. Jenner, "Civilization and Deodorization?," pp. 128–129. For positive remarks on Jorvik and its putative ability to "awaken" our senses, see Pocock, "The Senses in Focus," p. 13. For wise words on the need for rigorous contextualization in sensory history, especially in the context of material culture, see Classen, "Museum Manners."

9. http://www.amarillo.com/stories/062205/fri_2153161.shtml (accessed 2 December 2006).

10. For a more detailed explanation of how Civil War re-enactors try to recreate the sensate past, see my "Producing Sense, Consuming Sense, Making Sense."

11. On the historically situated meaning of visual evidence and abolitionism, see Clark, " 'The Sacred Rights of the Weak'." On color, see Pastoureau, *Blue*.

12. On acoustic shadows and Civil War sounds, see Ross, *Civil War Acoustic Shadows*; Mark M. Smith, "Of Bells, Booms, Sounds, and Silences."

13. Corbin, *Time, Desire, Horror*, 183. Note also Parr, "Notes for a More Sensuous History," 720; Carp, "Perception and Material Culture," p. 271.

14. Hoffer, *Sensory Worlds*, p. 14.

15. Herz, "Influence of Odors on Mood and Affective Cognition," pp. 160–177. On the gas liquid chromatographer, see Classen, Howes, Synnott, *Aroma*, pp. 198–200. On sugar and taste, see Mintz, *Sweetness and Power*.

16. Korsmeyer, "Introduction: Perspectives on Tastes," p. 3.

17. Revel, "Retrieving Tastes," pp. 51–53, quotations on pp. 51, 52; Mennell, "Of Gastronomes and Guides."

18. See Parr, "Notes for a More Sensuous History," pp. 721, 726, 743–745.

19. On McLuhan's work in this context, Howes, *Sensual Relations*, p. xxii; Howes, "Sensorial Anthropology," p. 186 (quotation). For a fascinating

etymological examination of intersensoriality, see Classen, *Worlds of Sense*, ch.3. Note too Marks, *The Unity of the Senses*. For very thoughtful work by art historians, see, for example, James, "Senses and Sensibility in Byzantium"; Phillips, "Making Sense Out of the Visual."

20. Abelson, *When Ladies Go A-Thieving*; Leach, "Transformations in a Culture of Consumption," pp. 324–326. Note also, Classen, *Worlds of Sense*, p. 6.

21. Mack, " 'Good Things to Eat in Suburbia'," pp. 15, 21–22, 28.

22. Mack, " 'Good Things to Eat in Suburbia'," pp. 3, 9–10.

23. Quoted in Mack, " 'Good Things to Eat in Suburbia'," pp. 26, 27.

24. Mack, " 'Good Things to Eat in Suburbia'," p. 45 (first quotation), p. 44 (second quotation).

25. Mack, " 'Good Things to Eat in Suburbia'," pp. 18–19. On the association between women, gustatory pleasure, and desire in Greek philosophy and its tenacious hold on the modern imagination, amply demonstrated here, see Korsmeyer, *Making Sense of Taste*, p. 5.

26. Mack, " 'Good Things to Eat in Suburbia'," pp. 20–25; Bowlby, *Carried Away*, pp. 35–36. The move toward quiet was reflected in architectural design and efforts to combat reverberation in the same period in the United States. See Thompson, *The Soundscape of Modernity*.

27. Gilman, *Goethe's Touch*, p. 1.

28. Rotter, *Comrades at Odds*, quotations, in order, on pp. 8, 9, 10, and see also p. 156.

29. On metaphor and the senses, see Mark M. Smith, *Listening to Nineteenth-Century America*, pp. 261–269; Hibbitts, "Making Sense of Metaphors." On race and smell, see my *How Race Is Made*; and my essay, "Making Scents Make Sense." On the senses in literature and text, see the various essays in Syrotinski and Maclachlan, eds., *Sensual Reading*; Parr, "Notes for a More Sensuous History," p. 742. On the global circulation of racial sensory stereotypes, see Gilroy, *Against Race*, pp. 35–46, 155–164. For powerful evidence of how the senses were used to mark and exploit a variety of immigrants to the United States, see Roediger, *Working Toward Whiteness*, pp. 51, 58, 79, 80, 85.

Bibliography

Abelson, Elaine S, *When Ladies Go A-Thieving: Middle-Class Shoplifters in the Victorian Department Store*, New York: Oxford University Press, 1989.
Ackerman, Diane, *A Natural History of the Senses*, New York: Vintage, 1991.
Agar, Jon, "Bodies, Machines and Noise," in Iwan Rhys Morus (ed.), *Bodies/Machines*, Oxford: Berg, 2002, pp. 197–220.
Alter, Nora M. and Koepnick, Lutz, "Introduction: Sound Matters," in Nora M. Alter and Lutz Koepnick (eds), *Sound Matters: Essays on the Acoustics of Modern German Culture*, Oxford: Berghahn Books, 2004, pp. 1–29.
Atkins, Keletso E., *The Moon Is Dead! Give Us Our Money! The Cultural Origins of an African Work Ethic, Natal, South Africa, 1843–1900*, Portsmouth, N.H.: Heinemann, 1993.
Attali, Jacques, *Noise: The Political Economy of Music*, Brian Maussumi (trans.), Minneapolis: University of Minnesota Press, 1985.
Barnes, David S., *The Great Stink of Paris and the Nineteenth-Century Struggle against Filth and Disease*, Baltimore, MD: Johns Hopkins University Press, 2006.
Baron, Lawrence, "Noise and Degeneration: Theodor Lessing's Crusade for Quiet," *Journal of Contemporary History* 17 (January 1982), pp. 165–178.
Bauman, Richard, *Let Your Words Be Few: Symbolism of Speaking and Silence Among Seventeenth-Century Quakers*, Cambridge: Cambridge University Press, 1983.
Beer, Gillian, "'Authentic Tidings of Invisible Things': Vision and the Invisible in the Later Nineteenth Century," in Teresa Brennan and Martin Jay (eds), *Vision in Context: Historical and Contemporary Perspectives on Sight*, New York: Routledge, 1996, pp. 83–98.
Bently, Lionel and Flynn, Leo (eds), *Law and the Senses: Sensational Jurisprudence*, London: Pluto Press, 1996.
Berger, John, *Ways of Seeing*, London: Penguin, 1972.
Berger, Martin A., *Sight Unseen: Whiteness and American Visual Culture*, Berkeley: University of California Press, 2005.
Blight, David W., "'Analyze the Sounds': Frederick Douglass' Invitation to Modern Historians of Slavery," in Stephan Palmié (ed.), *Slave Cultures and*

the Cultures of Slavery, Knoxville: University of Tennessee Press, 1995, pp. 1–11.

Bloch, Marc, *The Royal Touch: Monarchy and Miracles in France and England*, New York: Dorset Press, 1989.

Bouman, M. J., "Luxury and Control: The Urbanity of Street Lighting in Nineteenth-Century Cities," *Journal of Urban History* 14 (1987), pp. 7–37.

Bouman, M. J., "The 'Good Lamp is the Best Police' Metaphor and Ideologies of the Nineteenth-Century Urban Landscape," *American Studies*, 32 (1991), pp. 63–78.

Bourdieu, Pierre, "Taste of Luxury, Taste of Necessity," in Carolyn Korsmeyer (ed.), *The Taste Culture Reader: Experiencing Food and Drink*, Oxford: Berg, 2005, pp. 72–78.

Bowlby, Rachel, *Carried Away: The Invention of Modern Shopping*, New York: Columbia University Press, 2001.

Boyle, Marjorie O'Rourke, *Senses of Touch: Human Dignity and Deformity from Michelangelo to Calvin*, Leiden: Brill, 1998.

Brown, C. Mackenzie, "Purāna as Scripture: From Sound to Image of the Holy Word in the Hindu Tradition," *History of Religions* 26 (August 1986), pp. 68–86.

Brownlee, Peter, "The Economy of the Eyes: Vision and the Cultural Production of Market Revolution, 1800–1860," Ph.D. dissertation, George Washington University, 2003.

Bull, Michael and Back, Les (eds), *The Auditory Culture Reader*, Oxford: Berg, 2003.

Burke, Timothy, *Lifebuoy Men, Lux Women: Commodification, Consumption, and Cleanliness in Modern Zimbabwe*, Durham, NC: Duke University Press, 1996.

Burnett, Charles, "Perceiving Sound in the Middle Ages," in Mark M. Smith (ed.), *Hearing History: A Reader*, Athens, GA: University of Georgia Press, 2004, pp. 69–84.

Bynum, W. F. and Porter, Roy (eds), *Medicine and the Five Senses*, Cambridge: Cambridge University Press, 1993.

Camporesi, Piero, *The Anatomy of the Senses: Natural Symbols in Medieval and Early Modern Italy*, Allan Cameron (trans.), Cambridge: Polity Press, 1994.

Candlin, Fiona, "Don't Touch! Hands Off! Art, Blindness and the Conservation of Expertise," *Body and Society* 10 (2004), pp. 71–90.

Carp, Richard M., "Perception and Material Culture: Historical and Cross-Cultural Perspectives," *Historical Reflections/Reflexions Historiques* 23 (1997), pp. 269–300.

Carter, Paul, *The Sound In-Between: Voice, Space, Performance*, New South Wales: New South Wales University Press and New Endeavour Press, 1992.

Caseau, Béatrice, "The Use and Meaning of Fragrance in the Ancient World and their Christianization (100–900 AD)," Ph.D. dissertation, Princeton University, 1994.

Cherry, Deborah (ed.), *Art: History: Visual: Culture*, Malden, MA: Blackwell, 2005.
Chiang, Connie Y., "Monterey-by-the-Smell: Odors and Social Conflict on the California Coastline," *Pacific Historical Review* 73 (May 2004), pp. 183–214.
Chidester, David, *Word and Light: Seeing, Hearing, and Religious Discourse*, Urbana: University of Illinois Press, 1992.
Chidester, David, "The American Touch: Tactile Imagery in American Religion and Politics," in Constance Classen (ed.), *The Book of Touch*, Oxford: Berg, 2005, pp. 49–65.
Clark, Elizabeth B., "'The Sacred Rights of the Weak': Pain, Sympathy, and the Culture of Individual Rights in Antebellum America," *Journal of American History* 82 (September 1995), pp. 463–493.
Classen, Constance, "Sweet Colors, Fragrant Songs: Sensory Models of the Andes and the Amazon," *American Ethnologist* 17 (November 1990), pp. 722–735.
Classen, Constance, *Worlds of Sense: Exploring the Senses in History and Across Cultures*, New York: Routledge, 1993.
Classen, Constance, "Foundations for an Anthropology of the Senses," *International Social Science Journal* 153 (September 1997), pp. 401–412.
Classen, Constance, *The Color of Angels: Cosmology, Gender and the Aesthetic Imagination*, New York: Routledge, 1998.
Classen, Constance, "The Senses," in Peter N. Stearns (ed.), *Encyclopedia of European Social History From 1350–2000*, 4, New York: Gale, 2001, pp. 355–364.
Classen, Constance (ed.), *The Book of Touch*, Oxford: Berg, 2005.
Classen, Constance, "Fingerprints: Writing about Touch," in Constance Classen (ed.), *The Book of Touch*, Oxford: Berg, 2005, pp. 1–9.
Classen, Constance, "Feminine Tactics: Crafting and Alternative Aesthetics in the Eighteenth and Nineteenth Centuries," in Constance Classen (ed.), *The Book of Touch*, Oxford: Berg, 2005, pp. 228–239.
Classen, Constance, "Museum Manners: The Sensory Life of the Early Museum," *Journal of Social History* 40 (June 2007), pp. 895–914.
Classen, Constance and Howes, David, "The Museum as Sensescape: Western Sensibilities and Indigenous Artefacts," in Elizabeth Edwards, Chris Gosden, and Ruth Phillips (eds), *Sensible Objects: Colonialism, Museums and Material Culture*,. Oxford: Berg, 2006, pp. 199–222.
Classen, Constance , Howes, David, and Synnott, Anthony, *Aroma: The Cultural History of Smell*, New York: Routledge, 1994.
Coates, Peter A., "The Strange Stillness of the Past: Toward an Environmental History of Sound and Noise," *Environmental History* 10 (October 2005), pp. 636–665.
Cohen Bull, Cynthia Jean, "Sense, Meaning, and Perception in Three Dance Cultures," in Jane C. Desmond (ed.) *Meaning in Motion: New Cultural Studies of Dance*, Durham, NC: Duke University Press, 1997, pp. 269–287.

Connor, Steven, "The Modern Auditory I," in Roy Porter (ed.), *Rewriting the Self: Histories from the Renaissance to the Present*, London: Routledge, 1997, pp. 203–223.

Connor, Steven, *The Book of Skin*, Ithaca, NY: Cornell University Press, 2004.

Cook, James W., *The Arts of Deception: Playing with Fraud in the Age of Barnum*, Cambridge, MA: Harvard University Press, 2001.

Coolman, Boyd Taylor, *Knowing God by Experience: The Spiritual Senses in the Theology of William of Auxerre*, Washington, DC: Catholic University of America Press, 2004.

Corbin, Alain, *The Foul and the Fragrant: Odor and the French Social Imagination*, Miriam Kochan, Roy Porter, and Christopher Prendergast (trans.), Cambridge, MA: Harvard University Press, 1986.

Corbin, Alain, *Time, Desire and Horror: Towards a History of the Senses*, Jean Birrell (trans.), Cambridge: Polity Press, 1995.

Corbin, Alain, *Village Bells: Sound and Meaning in the 19th-Century French Countryside*, Martin Thom (trans.), New York: Columbia University Press, 1998.

Crary, Jonathan, *Techniques of the Observer: On Vision and Modernity in the Nineteenth Century*, Cambridge, MA: MIT Press, 1992.

Crowley, John E, *The Invention of Comfort: Sensibilities and Design in Early Modern Britain and Early America*, Baltimore, MD: Johns Hopkins University Press, 2001.

Cruz, Jon, *Culture on the Margins: The Black Spiritual and the Rise of American Cultural Interpretation*, Princeton, NJ: Princeton University Press, 1999.

Dalby, Andrew, *Dangerous Tastes: The Story of Spices*, Berkeley: University of California Press, 2000.

Damousi, Joy, "'The Filthy American Twang': Elocution, the Advent of American 'Talkies,' and Australian Cultural Identity," *American Historical Review* 112 (April 2007), pp. 394–416.

Daniel, E. Valentine, "The Pulse as an Icon in Siddha Medicine," in David Howes (ed.), *The Varieties of Sensory Experience: A Sourcebook in the Anthropology of the Senses*, Toronto: University of Toronto Press, 1991, pp. 100–110.

Das, Santanu, *Touch and Intimacy in First World War Literature*, New York: Cambridge University Press, 2005.

Davis, Susan G., "Touch the Magic," in *Uncommon Ground: Toward Reinventing Nature*, William Cronon (ed.), New York: Norton, 1995, pp. 207–217.

Davison, Graeme, *The Unforgiving Minute: How Australia Learned to Tell the Time*, New York: Oxford University Press, 1993.

Detienne, Marcel, *The Gardens of Adonis: Spices in Greek Mythology*, Janet Lloyd (trans.), Princeton, NJ: Princeton University Press, 1994.

Devereux, George, "Ethnopsychological Aspects of the Terms 'Deaf' and 'Dumb'," in David Howes (ed.) *Sensual Relations: Engaging the Senses in Culture and Social Theory*, Ann Arbor: University of Michigan Press, 2003, pp. 43–46.

Di Benedetto, Stephen, "Stumbling in the Dark: Facets of Sensory Perception and Robert Wilson's 'H.G.' Installation," *New Theatre Quarterly* 67 (2001), pp. 273–284.
Dohrn-van Rossum, Gerhard, *History of the Hour: Clocks and Modern Temporal Orders*, Chicago: University of Chicago Press, 1996.
Drobnick, Jim, "Reveries, Assaults and Evaporating Presences: Olfactory Dimensions in Contemporary Art," *Parachute* 89 (1998), pp. 10–19.
Drobnick, Jim (ed.), *Aural Cultures*, Toronto: YYZ Books, 2004.
Drobnick, Jim (ed.), *The Smell Culture Reader*, Oxford: Berg, 2006.
Eakin, Emily, "History You Can See, Hear, Smell, Touch, and Taste," *New York Times*, Saturday, December 20, 2003.
Eisenstein, Elizabeth L., *The Printing Press as an Agent of Change: Communications and Cultural transformations in Early Modern Europe*, Cambridge: Cambridge University Press, 1979.
Ekrich, A. Roger, *At Day's Close: Night in Times Past*, New York: Norton, 2005.
Elias, Norbert, *The History of Manners*, vol. 1: *The Civilizing Process*, Edmund Jephcott (trans.). New York, 1982.
Elkins, James, *The Object Stares Back: On the Nature of Seeing*, San Diego: Harvest, 1996.
Elkins, James, *Visual Studies: A Skeptical Introduction*, New York: Routledge, 2003.
Erlmann, Viet (ed.), *Hearing Cultures: Essays on Sound, Listening and Modernity*, Oxford: Berg, 2004.
Farquar, Judith, *Appetites: Food and Sex in Post-Socialist China*, Durham, NC: Duke University Press, 2002.
Farnell, Brenda, "Kinesthetic Sense and Dynamically Embodied Action," *Journal for the Anthropological Study of Human Movement*," 12 (2003), pp. 133–139.
Febvre, Lucien, *The Problem of Unbelief in the Sixteenth Century: The Religion of Rabelais*, Beatrice Gottlieb (trans.), Cambridge, MA: Harvard University Press, 1982.
Feld, Steven, *Sound and Sentiment: Birds, Weeping, Poetics and Song in Kaluli Expression*, Philadelphia: University of Pennsylvania Press, 1990.
Finnegan, Ruth, *Communicating: The Multiple Modes of Human Interconnection*, London: Routledge, 2002.
Finnegan, Ruth, "Tactile Communication," in Constance Classen (ed.), *The Book of Touch*, Oxford: Berg, 2005, pp. 18–25.
Fischer, Barbara, "Introduction," in Barbara Fischer (ed.), *Tasting Identities and Geographies in Art*, Toronto: YYZ Books, 1999, pp. 21–27.
Fisher, Jennifer, "Relational Sense: Towards a Haptic Aesthetics," *Parachute* 87 (Summer 1997), pp. 4–11.
Fisher, Jennifer, "Performing Taste," in Barbara Fischer (ed.), *Tasting Identities and Geographies in Art*, Toronto: YYZ Books, 1999, pp. 29–47.
Flint, Kate, *The Victorians and the Visual Imagination*, New York: Cambridge University Press, 2000.

Foucault, Michel, *The Birth of the Clinic: An Archaeology of Medical Perception*, A. M. Sheridan Smith (trans.), New York: Vintage Books, 1975.
Foucault, Michel, *Discipline and Punish: The Birth of the Prison*, Alan Sheridan (trans.), New York: Penguin, 1987.
Foucault, Michel, *The Order of Things: An Archaeology of the Human Sciences*, New York: Vintage Books, 1994.
Gabbacia, Donna R., "Colonial Creoles: The Formation of Tastes in Early America," in Carolyn Korsmeyer (ed.), *The Taste Culture Reader: Experiencing Food and Drink*, Oxford: Berg, 2005, pp. 79–85.
Gac, Scott, "Listening to the Progressives," *Reviews in American History* 32 (September 2004), pp. 407–412.
Garrioch, David, "Sounds of the City: The Soundscape of Early Modern European Towns," *Urban History* 30 (2003), pp. 6–26.
Garrioch, David, *The Making of Revolutionary France*, Berkeley: University of California Press, 2004.
Gay, Peter, *The Bourgeois Experience. Victoria to Freud. Volume 1. Education of the Senses*, New York: Oxford University Press, 1984.
Geaney, Jane, *On the Epistemology of the Senses in Early Chinese Thought*, Honolulu: University of Hawai'i Press, 2002.
Geller, Jay, "'A glance at the nose': Freud's Inscription of Jewish Difference," *American Imago* 49, no.4, pp. 427–444.
Gerth, Karl, "Commodifying Chinese Nationalism: MSG and the Flavor of Patriotic Production," in Susan Strasser (ed.), *Commodifying Everything: Relationships of the Market*, New York: Routledge, 2003, pp. 235–258.
Geurts, Kathryn Linn, *Culture and the Senses: Bodily Ways of Knowing in an African Community*, Berkeley: University of California Press, 2002.
Gigante, Denise, *Taste: A Literary History*, New Haven, CT: Yale University Press, 2005.
Gilman, Sander, *Goethe's Touch: Touching, Sexuality, and Seeing*, New Orleans: Graduate School of Tulane University, 1988.
Gilman, Sander, "Touch, Sexuality and Disease," in W. F. Bynum and Roy Porter (eds), *Medicine and the Five Senses*, Cambridge: Cambridge University Press, 1993, pp. 198–224.
Gilroy, Paul, *Against Race: Imagining Political Culture Beyond the Color Line*, Cambridge, MA: Belknap Press of Harvard University Press, 2000.
Gitelman, Lisa, *Scripts, Grooves, and Writing Machines: Representing Technology in the Edison Era*, Stanford, CA: Stanford University Press, 1999.
Godfrey, Sima, "Alain Corbin: Making Sense of French History," *French Historical Studies*, 25 (Spring 2002), pp. 381–398.
Goody, Jack, *The Logic of Writing and the Organization of Society*, Cambridge: Cambridge University Press, 1986.
Goody, Jack *The Interface between the Written and the Oral*, Cambridge: Cambridge University Press, 1987.

Goody, Jack, "The High and the Low: Culinary Culture in Asia and Europe," Carolyn Korsmeyer (ed.) in *The Taste Culture Reader: Experiencing Food and Drink*, Oxford: Berg, 2005, pp. 57–71.

Gorn, Elliot J., "'Gouge and bite, pull hair and scratch': The Social Significance of Fighting in the Southern Backcountry," *American Historical Review* 90 (1985), pp. 18–43.

Gouk, Penelope, "Some English Theories of Hearing in the Seventeenth Century: Before and After Descartes," in Charles Burnett, Michael Fend, and Penelope Gouk (eds), *The Second Sense: Studies in Hearing and Musical Judgement from Antiquity to the Seventeenth Century*, London: Warburg Institute, 1991, pp. 95–113.

Gouk, Penelope, "Raising Spirits and Restoring Souls: Early Modern Medical Explanations for Music's Effects", in Viet Erlmann (ed.), *Hearing Cultures: Essays on Sound, Listening and Modernity*, Oxford: Berg, 2004, pp. 87–105.

Gowing, Laura, *Common Bodies: Women, Touch and Power in Seventeenth-Century England*, New Haven, CT: Yale University Press, 2003.

Graham, Sandra Lauderdale, *House and Street: The Domestic World of Servants and Masters in Nineteenth-Century Rio de Janeiro*, Austin: University of Texas Press, 1992.

Grier, Katherine C., *Culture and Comfort: Parlor Making and Middle-Class Identity, 1850–1930*, Washington, DC: Smithsonian Institution Press, 1997.

Gronow, Jukka, "Champagne and Caviar: Soviet Kitsch," in Carolyn Korsmeyer (ed.), *The Taste Culture Reader: Experiencing Food and Drink*, Oxford: Berg, 2005, pp. 249–259.

Haden, Roger, "Taste in an Age of Convenience: From Frozen Food to Meals in 'the Matrix'," in Carolyn Korsmeyer (ed.), *The Taste Culture Reader: Experiencing Food and Drink*, Oxford: Berg, 2005, pp. 344–358.

Hall, Edward T., *The Hidden Dimension*, New York: Doubleday, 1969.

Hall, James, *The World as Sculpture: The Changing Status of Sculpture from the Renaissance to the Present*, London: Chatto and Windus, 1999.

Harvey, Elizabeth D, "Introduction: The Sense of All Senses," in Elizabeth D. Harvey (ed.), *Sensible Flesh: On Touch in Early Modern Culture*, Philadelphia: University of Pennsylvania Press, 2003, pp. 1–21.

Harvey, Susan Ashbrook, "St. Ephrem on the Scent of Salvation," *Journal of Theological Studies* 49 (April 1998), pp. 109–128.

Harvey, Susan Ashbrook, *Scenting Salvation: Ancient Christianity and the Olfactory Imagination*, Berkeley: University of California Press, 2006.

Head, Lynda, *Victorian Babylon: People, Streets and Images in Nineteenth-Century*, New Haven, CT: Yale University Press, 2000.

Herz, Rachel S., "Influence of Odors on Mood and Affective Cognition," in Catherine Rouby, et al. (ed.), *Olfaction, Taste, and Cognition*, Cambridge: Cambridge University Press, 2002, pp. 160–177.

Hibbitts, Bernard J., "Coming to Our Senses: Communication and Legal Expression in Performance Culture" 41 *Emory Law Journal* 4 (1992), pp. 874–959. Online version cited: http://www.law.pitt.edu/hibbitts/ctos.htm (accessed June 26, 2003).

Hibbitts, Bernard J., "Making Sense of Metaphors: Visuality, Aurality, and the Reconfiguration of American Legal Discourse," 16 *Cardozo Law Review* 229 (1994). Online version cited: http://www.law.pitt.edu/hibbitts/meta_int.htm (accessed January 15, 2000).

Hoffer, Peter Charles, *Sensory Worlds of Early America*, Baltimore, MD: Johns Hopkins University Press, 2004.

Houston, Stephen and Taube, Karl, "An Archaeology of the Senses: Perception and Cultural Expression in Ancient Mesoamerica," *Cambridge Archaeological Journal* 10 (2000), pp. 261–294.

Howes, David, "Scent and Sensibility," *Culture, Medicine and Psychiatry* 13 (1989), pp. 81–89.

Howes, David, "Controlling Textuality: A Call for a Return to the Senses," *Anthropologica* 33 (1990), pp. 55–73.

Howes, David, "Olfaction and Transition," in David Howes (ed.), *The Varieties of Sensory Experience: A Sourcebook in the Anthropology of the Senses*, Toronto: University of Toronto Press, 1991, pp. 128–147.

Howes, David, "Sensorial Anthropology," in David Howes (ed.), *The Varieties of Sensory Experience: A Sourcebook in the Anthropology of the Senses*, Toronto: University of Toronto Press, 1991, pp. 167–191.

Howes, David (ed.), *The Varieties of Sensory Experience: A Sourcebook in the Anthropology of the Senses*, Toronto: University of Toronto Press, 1991.

Howes, David, "The Senses in Medicine," *Culture, Medicine and Psychiatry* 19 (1995), pp. 125–133.

Howes, David, *Sensual Relations: Engaging the Senses in Culture and Social Theory*, Ann Arbor: University of Michigan Press, 2003.

Howes, David, "Introduction: 'To Summon All the Senses'," in David Howes (ed.), *Sensual Relations: Engaging the Senses in Culture and Social Theory*, Ann Arbor: University of Michigan Press, 2003, pp. 3–21.

Howes, David, "Forming Perceptions," in David Howes (ed.) *Empire of the Senses: The Sensual Culture Reader*, Oxford: Berg, 2005, pp. 399–402.

Howes, David, "Skinscapes: Embodiment, Culture, and Environment," in Constance Classen (ed.), *The Book of Touch*, Oxford: Berg, 2005, pp. 27–39.

Howes, David and Classen, Constance, "Sounding Sensory Profiles," in David Howes (ed.), *The Varieties of Sensory Experience: A Sourcebook in the Anthropology of the Senses*, Toronto: University of Toronto Press, 1991.

Howes, David and Lalonde, Marc, "The History of Sensibilities: Of the Standard of Taste In Mid-Eighteenth Century England and the Circulation of Smells in Post-Revolutionary France," *Dialectical Anthropology* 16 (1991), pp. 125–135.

Hunt, Alan, *Governance of the Consuming Passions: A History of Sumptuary Law*, New York: St. Martin's Press, 1996.

Ihde, Don, *Sense and Significance*, Pittsburgh: Duquesne University Press, 1973.
Informant 9F, "Russian Sensory Images," in Margaret Mead and Rhoda Métraux (eds), *The Study of Culture at a Distance*, Chicago: University of Chicago Press, 1953, pp. 162–169.
Irigaray, Luce, "This Sex Which Is Not One," in Elaine Marks and Isabelle de Courtivron (eds), *New French Feminisms: An Anthology*, Amherst: University of Massachusetts Press, 1980, pp. 99–106.
Irigaray, Luce, *Speculum of the Other Woman*, Gillian C. Hill (trans.), Ithaca, NY: Cornell University Press, 1985.
James, Liz, "Senses and Sensibility in Byzantium," in *Art: History: Visual: Culture*, Deborah Curry (ed.), Malden, MA: Blackwell, 2005, pp. 44–59.
Jay, Martin, "Scopic Regimes of Modernity," in Hal Foster (ed.), *Vision and Visuality*, Seattle, WA: Bay Press, 1988.
Jay, Martin, *Downcast Eyes: The Denigration of Vision in Twentieth-Century French Thought*, Berkeley: University of California Press, 1993.
Jenner, Mark S. R., "Civilization and Deodorization? Smell in Early Modern English Culture," in Peter Burke, Brian Harrison, and Paul Slack (eds), *Civil Histories: Essays Presented to Sir Keith Thomas*, New York: Oxford University Press, 2000, pp. 127–144.
Johnson, Geraldine A., "Touch, Tactility, and the Reception of Sculpture in Early Modern Italy," in Paul Smith and Carolyn Wilde (eds), *A Companion to Art Theory*, Malden, MA: Blackwell, 2002, pp. 61–74.
Johnson, James H., *Listening in Paris: A Cultural History*, Studies on the History of Society and Culture, 21, Berkeley CA: University of California Press, 1995.
Jonas, Hans, "The Nobility of Sight: A Study in the Phenomenology of the Senses," in *The Phenomenon of Life: Toward a Philosophical Biology*, New York: Harper and Row, 1966.
Jordanova, Ludmilla, "The Art and Science of Seeing in Medicine: Physiognomy 1780–1820," in W. F. Bynum and Roy Porter (eds), *Medicine and the Five Senses*, Cambridge: Cambridge University Press, 1993, pp. 122–133.
Jütte, Robert, *A History of the Senses: From Antiquity to Cyberspace*, James Lynn (trans.), Cambridge: Polity Press, 2005.
Kahn, Douglas, *Noise, Water, Meat: A History of Sound in the Arts*, Cambridge, MA: MIT Press, 1999.
Kahn, Douglas, "Sound Awake," *Australian Review of Books* (July 2000), pp. 21–22.
Kahn, Douglas, "Art and Sound," in Mark M. Smith (ed.), *Hearing History: A Reader*, Athens, GA: University of Georgia Press, 2004, pp. 36–50.
Keller, Eve, "The Subject of Touch: Medical Authority in Early Modern Midwifery," in Elizabeth D. Harvey (ed.), *Sensible Flesh: On Touch in Early Modern Culture*, Philadelphia: University of Pennsylvania Press, 2003, pp. 62–80.
Kemp, Martin, "'The Mark of Truth': Looking and Learning in some Anatomical Illustrations from the Renaissance and Eighteenth Century," in W. F. Bynum

and Roy Porter pp. (eds), *Medicine and the Five Senses*, Cambridge: Cambridge University Press, 1993, pp. 85–121.

Kern, Stephen, "Olfactory Ontology and Scented Harmonies: On the History of Smell," *Journal of Popular Culture* 4 (Spring 1974), pp. 816–824.

Korsmeyer, Carolyn, *Making Sense of Taste: Food and Philosophy*, Ithaca, NY: Cornell University Press, 1999.

Korsmeyer, Carolyn, "Introduction: Perspectives on Tastes," in Carolyn Korsmeyer (ed.), *The Taste Culture Reader: Experiencing Food and Drink*, Oxford: Berg, 2005, pp. 1–9.

Koslofsky, Craig, "Court Culture and Street Lighting in Seventeenth-Century Europe," *Journal of Urban History* 28 (September 2002), pp. 743–768.

Kurlansky, Mark, *Salt: A World History*, New York: Penguin, 2002.

Landes, David S., *Revolution in Time: Clocks and the Making of the Modern World*, Cambridge, MA: Harvard University Press, 1983.

Largey, Gale Peter and Watson, David Rodney, "The Sociology of Odors," *American Journal of Sociology* 77 (May 1972), pp. 1021–1034.

Lawrence, Susan C., "Educating the Senses: Students, Teachers and Medical Rhetoric in Eighteenth-Century London," in W. F. Bynum and Roy Porter (eds), *Medicine and the Five Senses*, Cambridge: Cambridge University Press, 1993, pp. 154–178.

Le Goff, Jacques, "Merchant's Time and Church's Time in the Middle Ages," in Jacques Le Goff, *Time, Work, and Culture in the Middle Ages*, Chicago: University of Chicago Press, 1980, pp. 29–42.

Le Goff, Jacques, "Labour Time in the 'Crisis' of the Fourteenth Century: From Medieval to Modern Time," in Jacques Le Goff, *Time, Work, and Culture in the Middle Ages*, Chicago: University of Chicago Press, 1980, pp. 43–52.

Leach, William R., "Transformations in a Culture of Consumption: Women and Department Stores, 1890–1925," *Journal of American History* 71 (September 1984), pp. 319–342.

Levin, David Michael (ed.), *Modernity and the Hegemony of Vision*, Berkeley: University of California Press, 1993.

Lowe, Donald, *History of Bourgeois Perception*, Chicago: University of Chicago Press, 1982.

Macinnis, Peter, *Bittersweet: The Story of Sugar*, Crows Nest, NSW, 2002.

McKitterick, David, *Print, Manuscript and the Search for Order 1450–1830*, Cambridge: Cambridge University Press, 2003.

McKnight, Brian E., "Sung Justice: Death by Slicing," *Journal of the American Oriental Society* 93 (July–September 1973), pp. 359–360.

McLuhan, Marshall, *The Gutenberg Galaxy* (University of Toronto Press, 1962.

McLuhan, Marshall, *Understanding Media: The Extensions of Man*, Cambridge, MA: MIT Press, 1994 [1964].

McWilliams, James E, *A Revolution in Eating: How the Quest for Food Shaped America*, New York: Columbia University Press, 2005.

Mack, Adam, "'Good Things to Eat in Suburbia': Supermarkets and American Consumer Culture, 1930–1970," Ph.D. dissertation, University of South Carolina, 2006.

Mandrou, Robert, *Introduction to Modern France, 1500–1640: An Essay in Historical Psychology*, R. E. Hallmark (trans.), New York: Holmes and Meier, 1976.

Marks, Lawrence E., *The Unity of the Senses: Interrelations among the Modalities*, New York: Academic Press, 1978.

Martland, Samuel Jefferson, "Progress Illuminating the World: Street Lighting in Santiago, Valparaiso and La Plata, 1840–1890," *Urban History* 29 (2002), pp. 223–238.

Martland, Samuel Jefferson, "Constructing Valparaiso: Infrastructure and the Politics of Progress in Chile's Port, 1842–1918," Ph.D. dissertation, University of Illinois at Urbana-Champaign, 2003.

Mennell, Stephen, "Of Gastronomes and Guides," in Carolyn Korsmeyer (ed.), *The Taste Culture Reader: Experiencing Food and Drink*, Oxford: Berg, 2005, pp. 239–248.

Meranze, Michel, "Michel Foucault, the Death Penalty and the Crisis of Historical Understanding," *Historical Reflections/Réflexions Historiques* 29 (2003), pp. 191–209.

Mintz, Sidney W., "Time, Sugar, and Sweetness," *Marxist Perspectives* 2 (Winter 1979/80), pp. 56–73.

Mintz, Sidney W., *Sweetness and Power: The Place of Sugar in Modern History*, New York: Viking, 1987.

Mintz, Sidney W., *Tasting Food, Tasting Freedom: Excursions into Eating, Culture, and the Past*, Boston: Beacon Press, 1996.

Morgan, Philip D., *Slave Counterpoint: Black Culture in the Eighteenth-Century Chesapeake and Lowcountry*, Chapel Hill: University of North Carolina Press, 1998.

Nead, Lynda. *Victorian Babylon: People, Streets and Images in Nineteenth-Century London*, New Haven, CT: Yale University Press, 2000.

Nicolson, Malcolm, "The Introduction of Percussion and Stethoscopy to Early Nineteenth-Century Edinburgh," in W. F. Bynum and Roy Porter (eds), *Medicine and the Five Senses*, Cambridge: Cambridge University Press, 1993, pp. 134–153.

Nutton, Vivian, "Galen at the Bedside: The Methods of a Medical Detective," in W. F. Bynum and Roy Porter (eds), *Medicine and the Five Senses*, Cambridge: Cambridge University Press, 1993, pp. 7–16.

Ong, Walter J., *The Presence of the Word*, New Haven, CT: Yale University Press, 1967.

Ong, Walter J., *Orality and Literacy: The Technologizing of the Word*, New York: Routledge, 1982.

Ong, Walter J., "The Shifting Sensorium," in David Howes (ed.), *The Varieties of Sensory Experience: A Sourcebook in the Anthropology of the Senses*, Toronto: University of Toronto Press, 1991, pp. 25–30.

Pallasmaa, Juhani, *The Eyes of the Skin: Architecture and the Senses*, London: Academy Editions, 1996.
Palmer, Richard, "In Bad Odor: Smell and its Significance in Medicine from Antiquity to the Seventeenth Century," in W. F. Bynum and Roy Porter (eds), *Medicine and the Five Senses*, Cambridge: Cambridge University Press, 1993, pp. 61–68.
Parr, Joy, "Notes for a More Sensuous History of Twentieth-Century Canada: The Timely, the Tacit, and the Material Body," *Canadian Historical Review* 82 (December 2001), pp. 720–745.
Parr, Joy, "Local Water Diversely Known: Walkerton Ontario, 200 and After," *Environment and Planning D: Society and Space* 22 (2004), pp. 1–18.
Pastoureau, Michel, *Blue: The History of a Color*, Princeton, NJ: Princeton University Press, 2001.
Payne, Matthew J., *Stalin's Railroad: Turksib and the Building of Socialism*, Pittsburgh: University of Pittsburgh Press, 2001.
Peters, J. C., *The Science & Art, or the Principles & Practice of Medicine*, New York: William Raddle, n.d.
Peterson, T. Sarah, *Acquired Taste: The French Origins of Modern Cooking*, Ithaca, NY: Cornell University Press, 1994.
Phillips, Ruth B., "Making Sense out/of the Visual: Aboriginal Presentations and Representations in Nineteenth-Century Canada," in Deborah Curry (ed.), *Art: History: Visual: Culture*, Malden, MA: Blackwell, 2005, pp. 113–135.
Picker, John M., "The Soundproof Study: Victorian Professionals, Work Space, and Urban Noise," *Victorian Studies* 42 (Spring 1999/2000), pp. 427–453.
Picker, John M,, *Victorian Soundscapes*, New York: Oxford University Press, 2003.
Pocock, Douglas, "The Senses in Focus," *Area* 25 (1993), pp. 11–16.
Porter, Roy, "The Rise of Physical Examination," in W. F. Bynum and Roy Porter (eds), *Medicine and the Five Senses*, Cambridge: Cambridge University Press, 1993, pp. 179–197.
Porter, Roy, *Flesh in the Age of Reason: The Modern Foundations of Body and Soul*, New York: W. W. Norton, 2003.
Price, Jennifer, "Looking for Nature at the Mall: A Field Guide to the Nature Company," in William Cronon (ed.), *Uncommon Ground: Toward Reinventing Nature*, New York: W. W. Norton, 1995, pp. 86–203.
Rath, Richard Cullen, *How Early America Sounded*, Ithaca, NY: Cornell University Press, 2003.
Reiser, Stanley J., "Technology and the Use of the Senses in Twentieth-Century Medicine," in W. F. Bynum and Roy Porter (eds), *Medicine and the Five Senses*, Cambridge: Cambridge University Press, 1993, pp. 262–273.
Revel, Jean-François, "Retrieving Tastes: Two Sources of Cuisine," in Carolyn Korsmeyer (ed.), *The Taste Culture Reader: Experiencing Food and Drink*, Oxford: Berg, 2005, pp. 51–56.
Ridley, Yvonne and Goodchild, Sophie, "Bare-knuckle is all the rage," *Independent*, Sunday, September 19, 1999, p. 3.

Riskin, Jessica, *Science in the Age of Sensibility: The Sentimental Empiricists of the French Enlightenment*, Chicago: University of Chicago Press, 2002.
Ritchie, Ian D., "The Nose Knows: Bodily Knowing in Isaiah 11.3," *Journal for the Study of the Old Testament* 87 (2000), pp. 59–73.
Rivlin, Robert and Gravelle, Karen, *Deciphering the Senses: The Expanding World of Human Perception*, New York: Simon and Schuster, 1985.
Rodaway, Paul, *Sensuous Geographies: Body, Sense and Place*, London: Routledge, 1994.
Roeder, George H., Jr, "Coming to Our Senses," *Journal of American History* 81 (December 1994), pp. 1112–1122.
Roediger, David R., *Working Toward Whiteness: How America's Immigrants Became White. The Strange Journey from Ellis Island to the Suburbs*, New York: Basic Books, 2005.
Rosen, Christine Meisner, "'Knowing' Industrial Pollution: Nuisance Law and the Power of Tradition in a Time of Rapid Economic Change, 1840–1864," *Environmental History* 8 (October 2003), pp. 565–597.
Rosenthal, Angela, "*Visceral* Culture: Blushing and the Legibility of Whiteness in Eighteenth-Century British Portraiture," in Deborah Curry (ed.), *Art: History: Visual: Culture*, Malden, MA: Blackwell, 2005, pp. 85–112.
Ross, Charles D., *Civil War Acoustic Shadows*, Shippensburg, PA: White Mane, 2001.
Rotter, Andrew J., *Comrades at Odds: The United States and India, 1947–1964*, Ithaca, NY: Cornell University Press, 2000.
Rudy, Gordon, *Mystical Language of Sensation in the Later Middle Ages*, New York: Routledge, 2002.
Schafer, R. Murray, *The Soundscape: Our Sonic Environment and the Tuning of the World*, Rochester, VT: Inner Traditions, 1994.
Schivelbusch, Wolfgang, *Disenchanted Night: The Industrialization of Light in the Nineteenth Century*, Berkeley: University of California Press, 1988.
Schivelbusch, Wolfgang, *Tastes of Paradise: A Social History of Spices, Stimulants, and Intoxicants*, David Jacobson (trans.), New York: Vintage Books, 1992.
Schmidt, Leigh Eric, *Hearing Things: Religion, Illusions, and the American Enlightenment*, Cambridge, MA: Harvard University Press, 2000.
Sen, Satadru, "The Imperial Touch: Schooling Male Bodies in Colonial India, Part II," in Constance Classen (ed.), *The Book of Touch*, Oxford: Berg, 2005, pp. 171–176.
Smilor, Raymond, "Cacophony at 34th and 6th: The Noise Problem in America, 1900–1930," *American Studies*, 18 (1977), pp. 23–38.
Smilor, Raymond, "Confronting the Industrial Environment: The Noise Problem in America, 1893–1932," Ph.D. dissertation, University of Texas, 1978.
Smilor, Raymond, "Personal Boundaries in the Urban Environment: The Legal Attack on Noise: 1865–1930," *Environmental Review*, 3 (1979), pp. 24–36.
Smilor, Raymond, "Toward an Environmental Perspective: The Anti-Noise Campaign, 1883–1932," in Martin V. Melosi (ed.), *Pollution and Reform in*

American Cities, 1870–1930, Austin: University of Texas Press, 1980, pp. 135–151.

Smith, Bruce R., *The Acoustic World of Early Modern England: Attending to the O-Factor*, Chicago: University Press of Chicago, 1999.

Smith, Jeffrey Chipps, *Sensuous Worship: Jesuits and the Art of the Early Catholic Reformation in Germany*, Princeton, NJ: Princeton University Press, 2002.

Smith, Mark M., "Old South Time in Comparative Perspective," *American Historical Review* 101 (December 1996), pp. 1432–1469.

Smith, Mark M., *Listening to Nineteenth-Century America*, Chapel Hill: University of North Carolina Press, 2001.

Smith, Mark M., "Of Bells, Booms, Sounds, and Silences: Listening to the Civil War South," in Joan Cashin (ed.), *The War Was You and Me: Civilians and the American Civil War*, Princeton, NJ: Princeton University Press 2002, pp. 9–34.

Smith, Mark M., "Making Sense of Social History," *Journal of Social History* 37 (1, Fall 2003), pp. 165–186.

Smith, Mark M. (ed.), *Hearing History: A Reader*, Athens, GA: University of Georgia Press, 2004.

Smith, Mark M., "Introduction: Onward to Audible Pasts," in Mark M. Smith (ed.), *Hearing History: A Reader*, Athens, GA: University of Georgia Press, 2004.

Smith, Mark M., "Making Scents Make Sense: White Noses, Black Smells, and Desegregation," in Peter Stearns (ed.), *American Behavioral History*, New York: New York University Press, 2005, pp. 179–198.

Smith, Mark M., *How Race Is Made: Slavery, Segregation, and the Senses*, Chapel Hill: University of North Carolina Press, 2006.

Smith, Mark M., "Producing Sense, Consuming Sense, Making Sense: Perils and Prospects for Sensory History," *Journal of Social History* 40 (June 2007), 841–858.

Smith, Mark M., "The Skin-Man: Getting in Touch with Abraham Lincoln," (Work in progress: in author's possession).

Smith, Roger, "Self-Reflection and the Self," in Roy Porter (ed.), *Rewriting the Self: Histories from the Renaissance to the Present*, London and New York: Routledge, 1997, pp. 49–57.

Smith, Shawn Michelle, *American Archives: Gender, Race, and Class in Visual Culture*, Princeton, NJ: Princeton University Press, 1999.

Smith, Shawn Michelle, *Photography on the Color Line: W. E. B. Du Bois, Race, and Visual Culture*, Durham, NC: Duke University Press, 2004.

Smith, Susan J., "Beyond Geography's Visible Worlds: A Cultural Politics of Music," *Progress in Human Geography* 21 (1997), pp. 501–529.

Stallybrass, Peter, "Marx's Coat," in Patricia Spyer (ed.), *Border Fetishisms: Material Objects in Unstable Places*, New York: Routledge, 1998.

Stallybrass, Peter and Allon White, "Bourgeois Perception: The Gaze and the Contaminating Touch," in Constance Classen (ed.), *The Book of Touch*, Oxford: Berg, 2005, pp. 289–291.

Starn, Randolph, "Seeing Culture in a Room for a Renaissance Prince," in Lynn Hunt (ed.), *The New Cultural History*, Berkeley: University of California Press, 1989, pp. 205–232.

Sterne, Jonathan, *The Audible Past: Cultural Origins of Sound Reproduction*, Durham, NC: Duke University Press, 2003.

Stevens, Scott Manning, "New World Contacts and the Trope of the 'Naked Savage'," in Elizabeth D. Harvey (ed.), *Sensible Flesh: On Touch in Early Modern Culture*, Philadelphia: University of Pennsylvania Press, 2003, pp. 125–140.

Steward, Jill and Alexander Cowan (eds), *The City and the Senses: Urban Culture Since 1550*, Aldershot: Ashgate, 2007.

Stewart, Susan, "Prologue: From the Museum of Touch," in Marius Kwint, Christopher Breward, and Jeremy Aynsley (eds), *Material Memories*, Oxford: Berg, 1999, pp. 17–36.

Stoller, Paul, "Sound in Songhay Cultural Experience," *American Ethnologist* 11 (1984), pp. 559–570.

Stoller, Paul, *Sensuous Scholarship*, Philadelphia: University of Pennsylvania Press, 1997.

Sui, Daniel Z., "Visuality, Aurality, and Shifting Metaphors of Geographical Thought in the Late Twentieth Century," *Annals of the Association of American Geographers* 90 (2000), pp. 322–343.

Sutton, David, "Sensory Memory and the Construction of 'Worlds'," *Remembrance of Repasts: An Anthropology of Food and Memory*, Oxford: Berg, 2001, 73–102.

Sutton, David, "Listen to that Scent! Travelling Tastes and Smells Among Greek Immigrants," *Detours Online Magazine*, 5 (May 2003). Online at http://www.prairie.org/index.cfm/fuseaction/dir_resources.detours_page/page_id/8eae10a8-1774-43ac-a15b-fd555fd338d6/object_id/b20af54e-7c32-43febf4a- df4dac542399/ListentothatScent.cfm (accessed 4/6/2005).

Swislocki, Mark S., "Feast and Famine in Republican Shanghai: Urban Food Culture, Nutrition, and the State," Ph.D. dissertation, Stanford University, 2002.

Synnott, Anthony, "Puzzling over the Senses: From Plato to Marx," in David Howes (ed.), *The Varieties of Sensory Experience: A Sourcebook in the Anthropology of the Senses*, Toronto: University of Toronto Press, 1991, pp. 61–76.

Synnott, Anthony, "A Sociology of Smell," *Canadian Review of Sociology and Anthropology* 28 (November 1991), pp. 437–459.

Synnott, Anthony, *The Body Social: Symbolism, Self and Society*, London: Routledge, 1993.

Synnott, Anthony, "Handling Children: To Touch or Not to Touch?," in Constance Classen (ed.), *The Book of Touch*, Oxford: Berg, 2005, pp. 41–47.

Syrotinski, Michael and Ian Maclachlan (eds), *Sensual Reading: New Approaches to Reading in Its Relations to the Senses*, Lewisburg, PA: Bucknell University Press, 2001.

Theweleit, Klaus, "Sexuality and the Drill: The Body Reconstructed in the Military Academy," in Constance Classen (ed.), *The Book of Touch*, Oxford: Berg, 2005, pp. 178–185.

Thomas, Keith, "Magical Healing: The King's Touch," in Constance Classen (ed.), *The Book of Touch*, Oxford: Berg, 2005, 354–362.
Thompson, E. P., "Rough Music," *Customs in Common*, London: New Press, 1991, 467–538.
Thompson, Emily, *The Soundscape of Modernity: Architectural Acoustics and the Culture of Listening in America, 1900–1933*, Cambridge, MA: MIT Press, 2002.
Toporkov, Andrei, "The Devil's Candle? Street Lighting," *History Today* 46 (November 1996), pp. 34–36.
Tuan, Yi-Fu, "The Pleasures of Touch," in Constance Classen (ed.), *The Book of Touch*, Oxford: Berg, 2005, pp. 74–79.
Tyndale-Biscoe, C. E., "The Imperial Touch: Schooling Male Bodies in Colonial India, Part I," in Constance Classen (ed.), *The Book of Touch*, Oxford: Berg, 2005, pp. 168–170.
Vazsonyi, Nicholas, "Hegemony Through Harmony: German Identity, Music, and Enlightenment around 1800," in Nora M. Alter and Lutz Koepnick (eds), *Sound Matters: Essays on the Acoustics of Modern German Culture*, Oxford: Berghahn Books, 2004, pp. 33–48.
Vernant, J.-P., "Introduction," in Marcel Detienne, *The Gardens of Adonis: Spices in Greek Mythology*, Janet Lloyd (trans.), Princeton, NJ: Princeton University Press, 1994, pp. vii–xli.
Vinge, Louise, *The Five Senses: Studies in a Literary Tradition*, Lund: CWK Gleerup, 1975.
Walker, Daniel, *No More, No More: Slavery and Cultural Resistance in Havana and New Orleans*, Minneapolis: University of Minnesota Press, 2004.
White, Shane and White, Graham, "'I was nearly stunned by the noise he made': Listening to African American Religious Sound in the Era of Slavery," *American Nineteenth Century History*, 1 (Spring 2000), pp. 34–61.
White, Shane and White, Graham, *The Sounds of Slavery: Discovering African American History through Songs, Sermons, and Speech*, Boston: Beacon, 2005.
Wober, Mallory, "Sensotypes," *Journal of Social Psychology* 70 (October 1966), pp. 181–189.
Wolfson, Elliot R., *Through a Speculum That Shines: Vision and Imagination in Medieval Jewish Mysticism*, Princeton, NJ: Princeton University Press, 1994.
Woolf, D. R., "Speech, Text, and Time: The Sense of Hearing and the Sense of the Past in Renaissance England," *Albion* 18 (1986), pp. 159–193.
Zakim, Michael, *Ready-Made Democracy: A History of Men's Dress in the American Republic, 1760–1860*, Chicago: University of Chicago Press, 2003.

Index

acoustemology, 22, 47
acoustic shadows, 121–2
Acquired Immune Deficiency
  Syndrome (AIDS), 110
Adorno, Theodor, 49
Africa, 2
  alleged odors of, 73
  colonization of, 56, 83
  drum languages of, 46
  and proximate senses, 137n19
  and sensory relationship to
    technology, 8–9
  and taste, 84–5
African Americans, 122
  and alleged odor of, 71–2, 131
  and aural acuity, 51
  history of, 5
Age of Reason, 31, 32
  see also Enlightenment
Albany, GA, 35–6
Alberti, Leon Battista, 23, 140n9
Alter, Nora M., 50
American Civil War, 8, 49, 69, 102, 106, 121–2
American Revolution, 85, 107
Annales School, 6–7
Anne (Queen), 105
Aquinas, Thomas, 28–9
architecture, 28, 43, 54, 94, 113, 140n9
Argentina, 38
Aristotle, 28, 44, 76, 93
Ashmolean Museum, 115

Attali, Jacques, 41–2
aurality, 6, 41
  and colonialism, 56, 59
  during the Enlightenment, 33–4, 41
  during the Middle Ages, 44
  and identity politics, 49
  and modernity, 48, 57–9
  and non-literate societies, 46
  and orality, 9–10, 22
  as religious expression, 52
  and silence, 42, 50–3, 128
  and soundscapes, 22, 44–5, 49, 51, 54, 121, 128, 136n10
Australia, 2, 57
Avicenna, 65

Bacon, Francis, 63
ballet, 23–4, 114
Barnes, David S., 67
Barthes, Roland, 20
bells, 7, 43–5, 48–9, 56–7, 122
Bentham, Jeremy, 26
Berenson, Bernard, 113
Bernard of Clairvaux, 98–9
blackness, 37, 72, 110, 153n41
  see also African Americans; race
Bonaventure, 98
boxing, 102, 111
breast-feeding, 112
British Museum, 115
Burnett, Charles, 44
Bynum, W. F., 7, 135n10

173

Calcutta, 69
Calvin, John, 64
Candlin, Fiona, 115
capitalism, 47, 66, 73, 84
  association with sight, 19, 23, 139n32
  aurality of, 49, 53, 56
  tactility of, 95, 115
  and taste, 127
Carter, Paul, 57
Caseau, Béatrice, 61
Catholic Reformation, 64
Cavendish, Mary, 32
Cézanne, Paul, 114
Chapman, Edmund, 100
Charles II, 104–5
Chauncy, Charles, 52
Chesapeake, VA, 46
Chiang, Connie Y., 70–1
Chiang, Kai-shek, 88
Chidester, David, 95, 105
Chile, 38, 69
China, 2, 29, 70, 77–8, 87–90, 106, 150n30
Christianity, 28, 51–2, 62–4, 78–9, 97
Chrysostom, John, 28
class and classes, 7, 24, 67
  and aurality, 45, 48–9, 51, 53
  distinctions among, 15, 26, 59, 65–6, 78, 86, 108
  emergence of, 1, 18, 90
  and hygiene, 71
  interests of, 16
  intersection with gender, 16, 18, 60, 77, 95, 101
  and smells, 66, 69
  social instability of, 34–5
  and taste, 75, 82, 88–90
  and touching, 101, 106–8
Classen, Constance, 7
  and aurality, 46
  and the church, 24
  and critique of occularcentrism, 12–13, 20–1, 32, 65, 93, 114–15
  and cultural construction of senses, 3, 16, 118, 133n3–4, 135n10, 138n28
  and olfactory senses, 59, 63, 65
  and orality, 138n22

cleanliness, 23, 64–6, 68, 70, 77, 111, 126, 153n41
clocks, 56–7
clothing, 71, 82, 103, 104, 106, 107
Colonial Williamsburg, 119–21
colonialism, 1
  aurality of, 56–7, 59
  sights of, 139n32
  smell of, 65, 68, 72, 73, 119
  tactility of, 96–7, 105, 110, 111
Columbus, Christopher, 110
commodities, 75, 83–4, 88, 115–16
communism, 23, 73, 88
Connor, Steven, 20
consumerism, 5
consumption, 116–17, 121
  and class, 82
  culture of, 126–8
  of food, 87, 88, 90
  and law, 75, 77
  of sugar, 84, 85
Constable, John, 113
Continental Congress (U.S.), 107
Cooee, 57
cooking, 72, 79, 80, 85, 87
comfort, 95, 103–4, 108, 127
Corbin, Alain, 136n11
  and aurality, 48–9
  and history of smell, 7, 67–8, 108–9
  and sensory construction, 15–16, 122
crime, 26, 38, 67
Crooke, Helkiah, 44
Crowley, John, 103, 135–6n10
Cubists, 114

Daniel, E. Valentine, 48
de Lille, Alain, 97
de Montaigne, Michel, 27, 64
Defoe, Daniel, 104
democracy, 16, 49, 51, 52, 105–8
Derrida, Jacques, 20
Descartes, René, 31
Devereux, George, 47
Diderot, Denis, 31
diet, 77–8, 82, 84–6, 88–90, 124
diplomatic history, 5, 130, 131
discomfort, 49, 103–4

disease
 aural association with, 43
 and blackness, 153n41
 and smelling, 60, 65, 67–8, 71–3
 and tactility, 99–100, 108–12
 visual association with, 34
Domesday Book, 43
Dublin, 45
Duden, Barbara, 118

ears, 4, 9, 11–12, 22, 47, 52, 55, 57, 122, 125
Edward the Confessor, 105
Engels, Friedrich, 107
England, 24, 42–4, 79, 82–3, 100, 104–7, 112
Elias, Norbert, 6, 102
Enlightenment, 1, 31–2, 34, 48, 52, 96
 in America, 6, 13, 103
 and aurality, 41, 50
 and olfaction, 59, 63
 privileging of seeing, 9, 14, 17–20, 21, 28, 31, 48, 52, 58, 63, 65, 81, 100, 114, 141n21
 and tasting, 81, 90
 and touching, 95, 100, 102
eroticism, 94, 127
ethnicity, 60, 73, 87, 130
eyes, 9, 11, 61, 68, 102, 107, 126
 and art, 113–15
 Enlightenment concepts of, 14
 and Foucault, 26
 and historiography, 20–1
 privileging of, 28–31
 and race, 37
 and technologies, 33, 35
Ezra, Ibn, 61

Febvre, Lucien, 6, 67
Feld, Steven, 47
Ferguson, John H., 36
Flagellent Movement, 97
Flint, Kate, 34, 142n31
food, 73, 75–91, 119–21, 124–5, 127
Foucault, Michel, 6–7, 25–6, 67
France, 6, 14–15, 48–9, 67, 84, 90, 96, 108, 126

Gabaccia, Donna R., 85
Galen, 43, 60, 65, 75, 96, 141n21
gas liquid chromatographer, 123
Gay, Peter, 112
gaze, 15, 23, 25, 33, 48, 95, 115
Geaney, Jane, 29–30
gender, 1, 5
 and intersection with class, 16, 26, 60, 65, 70, 74, 95
 and intersection with race, 21, 60, 65, 70, 74, 75, 95
 and modernity, 18
 sensory components of, 33, 70, 74, 76, 136n12
 and sight, 21, 32
 tactility of, 96, 109
 and taste, 77, 85, 127
 and violence, 99–100
Germany, 50, 53, 64, 96
Gerth, Karl, 88
gestures, 4, 12, 22, 93, 103, 105
Ghiberti, Lorenzo, 113–14
Gilman, Sander, 94–5, 99, 110, 129, 153n41
Gitelman, Lisa, 55
Gouk, Penelope, 44
Gowing, Laura, 101
great divide theory, 17, 21–2, 38, 128
 and Foucault, 6
 and McLuhan and Ong, 8, 10–15, 31–3
 and orality, 41
Greece, 43, 60, 75, 77, 79, 87, 88

Hadewijch of Brabant, 98–9
hands, 96–7, 100–2, 104–9, 111–12
hapticity, *see* skin; touching
Harvey, Elizabeth D., 103–4
Harvey, Susan Ashbrook, 62
hearing, 1, 4, 6, 8, 18, 41, 59, 133n4
 as bridge between other senses, 41, 45
 and class, 24, 45–46, 103
 and colonialism, 56
 commodification of, 127
 inaccuracy of, 44
 and modernity, 48–56
 privileging of, 10, 23, 28–9, 32, 42–3, 47, 76

and racial identity, 55
and religious expression, 13, 46, 51–2, 64, 98
as segregation tool, 37
and sight, 9
and speech, 9
Hebrews, 6, 76
Hibbitts, Bernard, 11–12, 22, 42, 96, 137n16
Hoffer, Charles Peter, 118–19, 121–3, 124
Holt, L. E., 112
Howes, David, 125, 134n6, 135n10, 138n22
  and critique of visual privileging, 19, 20–1, 23, 137n19
  and Foucault, 7
  and McLuhan and Ong, 8, 10–12
  and smell, 59
  and tactility, 81–3, 114
Hughes, Robert, 113
humanism, 110
Hume, David, 81–3
Hunt, Alan, 16
hygiene, 71, 73

imperialism, 1, 18, 47, 56–7, 65, 82, 88, 109–11
Incas, 30, 46
India, 69, 130
Indochina, 47
industrialization, 1, 18, 26, 52, 66
intersensorality, 12, 16, 29, 118, 125–8
Islam, 79, 80, 90

Jameson, Anna, 24
Jay, Martin, 20, 114, 138n27
Jenner, Mark S. R., 17, 65
Jesuits, 64–5
Jesus Christ, 25, 62, 63, 78, 97–8, 124
Jews, 61–2, 141n22
Johns Hopkins University Press, 123
Johnson, Geraldine A., 113
Johnson, James H., 50–1
Jorvik, 120–2
Jutte, Robert, 5, 14, 115, 118–119, 134n5

Kahn, Douglas, 42, 134n6, 144n3
Kaluli, 47–8
Kant, Immanuel, 81, 100
Kashmiri Pandit students, 111
kissing, 96, 97, 112, 113
Koepnick, Lutz, 50
Korsmeyer, Carolyn, 75–6, 124, 138n30

labor, 90
  and aurality, 56
  manual, 68, 108–9
  mental, 53
  and odor, 66, 71–3
  and sight, 33
  and slavery, 51, 106
  and tactility, 48–9
  and taste, 83
  wage, 51, 56, 106
Lacan, Jacques, 20
Laënnec, René-Théophile-Hyacinthe, 48
Lalonde, Marc, 7, 81–3
legal history, 7, 11, 136n12
Levin, David Michael, 21
Lewis, C.S., 93
Lincoln, Abraham, 106
London, 34–5, 45, 53, 65, 100, 107
Louisiana, 36–7
Lowe, Donald, 21
Luther, Martin, 64

Mack, Adam, 126–7
Magnus, Albertus, 44
Malay, 47
Mandrou, Robert, 6
manners, 6, 102, 108
Martland, Samuel, 38
Marx, Karl, 14, 16, 138n25
masculinity, 23, 76, 101, 106–7, 109, 111, 113
masturbation, 112
Maya, 30
McLuhan, Marshall, 136n10, 137n19
  and aurality, 22, 41–2, 138n22
  and great divide theory, 8, 10–15, 31–3
  and intersensorality, 16–17
  privileging of sight, 27, 125

McWilliams, James E., 86
medicine, 7, 118, 133n2, 136n11
  and aurality, 43, 48
  and importance of sight, 24, 33, 100, 141n21
  and smell, 60, 79, 123
  and tactility, 94, 96
Merleau-Ponty, Maurice, 20
Mesopotamia, 96
Michelangelo, 113
migration, 74, 124
Mintz, Sidney W., 84
Molyneux's Problem, 31
monosodium glutamate (MSG), 87–8
Moscow, 45
Mozart, Wolfgang Amadeus, 50
murder, 15, 95
museums, 115–16, 117, 119, 123
music, 41–3, 50, 53, 55–6, 74, 121, 144n3
mythologies, 28, 61–2, 76

nakedness, 110
nationalism, 1, 48–9, 82, 87–8, 130
Native Americans, 56, 84–5, 105, 110–11, 122
Nature Company, 116
Nazis, 50
noise, 42–3, 45, 121–3, 136n12
  as component of Aurality, 48–50
  and modernity, 57, 68–9, 128
  negative associations with, 8, 52–4, 71
  as transgression, 25, 27
Noise Abatement Commission (NY), 54
noses, 26, 70, 73, 123, 125, 130
  as arbiter of class, 66, 68
  as arbiter of race, 37, 72
  medical uses, 60–1
  and religious practice, 63
  role in transgression, 28
  and tourism, 120

occularcentrism, see sight, privileging of

O'Connor, Fergus, 107
odors, 17, 27, 130
  as arbiter of race, 60–1, 131
  and disease, 65–7
  and religious practice, 25, 61
  subjectivity of, 70–3
olfaction, see smelling
Ong, Walter
  and aurality, 22, 41–2, 138n22
  and great divide theory, 8, 10–11, 13, 14
  and intersensorality, 16–17
  privileging of sight, 27
oral-aural societies, 9–10
Origen of Alexander, 97–8
Orwell, George, 66
ownership, 25, 57, 96, 114–16

paganism, 62–3
pain, 8, 76, 95, 97–8, 105
Paine, Thomas, 107
Panopticon, 25–6
Paris, 68, 69
Parr, Joy, 23, 50, 90–1, 94, 135n10
Pastoureau, Michel, 121
perfume, 60–6, 68, 72, 77, 109
Peterson, T. Sarah, 79–80
photography, 20, 24, 26, 34, 36
Pinel, Philippe, 31
pleasure, 28, 62, 63, 76, 79, 89, 97, 108, 112, 127
Plato, 28–9, 43, 76, 93
Plessy v. Ferguson, 36–7
Plessy, Homer, 36–7
pollution, 68, 99, 110
Polo, Marco, 77
Pope, Alexander, 81
Porter, Roy, 7, 32
possession, 30, 101, 114–6
premodern societies, 41–2, 98, 118
  and noise, 53
  privileging of sight, 17–18, 27–8, 33, 100, 141n21
  and proximate senses, 2–3, 97
  and sexuality, 128–9
  and smell, 37, 59, 83, 120
  and sumptuary laws, 16
  and tactility, 31, 33, 95–6, 102

print revolution, 27
  and hearing, 44, 46, 58–9
  historical importance of, 11–12, 31, 33
  and privileging of sight, 2, 10, 16, 18, 21, 32, 58, 125
  and religious practice, 25, 29
  and tactility, 93, 125
private space, 67, 72
Progressive Era, 53
prostitution, 35, 66
Protestant Reformation, 24–5, 63, 110
proximate senses, *see* smelling, tasting and touching
public space, 25, 35, 61, 72
Puritans, 64, 105

Quakers, 105

race, 73, 75, 83
  and consumerism, 55
  and hearing, 55
  instability of, 35–7
  and modernity, 18, 27, 35, 110
  and racism, 70
  and sensory history, 1, 5, 21
  and sight, 21, 55
  and slavery, 109
  and smell, 60, 65, 70–2, 74, 143n39
  and tactility, 95
Rath, Richard, 22, 45–6
recorded sound, 55
religious space, 43
Renaissance, 13, 23, 48
  and print revolution, 31, 48, 58
  privileging of seeing, 9–10, 19, 22, 28, 31–3
  and tasting, 80
  and touching, 99, 102, 110, 113–14
Restoration, 105
Revel, Jean-François, 124
Rio de Janeiro, 69, 71
Riskin, Jessica, 31
Ritchie, Ian D., 61
Roeder, George H., 7–8

Rome (Ancient), 42–3, 60–2, 64, 77, 79–80, 125
Rotter, Andrew J., 130
Rudy, Gordon, 97–9, 152n15
Russia, 37–8, 73–4, 90

St. Ephrem, 62
St. Ignatius, 29, 64, 78, 97
Sartre, Jean-Paul, 20
Schafer, R. Murray, 22, 136n10
Schmidt, Leigh Eric, 6, 13, 51–2
scent, 59, 63, 74
  as cultural markers, 61, 73, 120, 123
  gendering of, 66, 109
  marginalization of, 29, 68
  racial associations of, 27, 72
  and religious practice, 62–3
  and status, 30, 60, 70
science, 23, 25, 31–2, 48, 67, 80
Sea World, 116
Second World War, 112, 123, 126–7
seeing
  and association with logic, 10, 23, 25, 34, 36, 93
  and aurality, 45, 55, 63, 76
  and conceptions of self, 27
  consumption of, 126–7
  distortions of, 35
  and gender, 21
  and history of, 1, 5, 19–21, 38
  instability of, 55
  as a lesser sense, 28, 115
  and modernity, 27, 38, 95
  privileging of, 8, 15, 19–21, 23, 25, 27–8, 33, 44, 48, 65
  and race, 21, 37, 55
  reliability of, 35
  and technology, 126
  and touching, 99–100
  in Victorian England, 35
segregation, 35–7, 50, 72
selfhood, 1, 20, 27, 47, 65–7, 98, 102, 110
senses, *see* aurality, seeing, smelling, tasting, and touching
sensory space, 27

sensory history, 11, 16, 20, 29, 93–4, 117–9, 125–31, 134n6, 135n10
sensory stereotypes, 17, 72, 112, 127, 130–1
sensualism, 24–5, 63–4, 79–80, 112, 127
sewer systems, 26, 34–5, 69, 130
sexuality, 128
   gendering of, 66, 97
   and race, 110, 153n41
   and religious practice, 76
   and tactility, 94, 99–101, 112
Shaffer, Wade, 120–1
Siddha, 96–97
silence, *see* aurality, and silence
skin, 94–5, 103, 104, 107, 113, 114, 116, 125
   and class, 101–2, 103, 108, 112
   gendering of, 96, 101, 106
   and medicine, 24, 61
   and race, 37, 55, 71, 109–10, 111
   and religious practice, 28, 97
slavery, 47, 49, 51, 53, 71, 85, 106, 109
smelling, 1, 2, 3, 7–8, 23, 41, 118
   association with disease, 34–5, 60–1, 65, 68, 141n21
   association with taste, 18
   and class, 66–7, 71
   consumption of, 119–21, 127
   and cuisine, 70, 73
   as generator of knowledge, 7
   history of, 59, 65, 133–4n4
   and industrialization, 67–9
   and masculinity, 77
   and modernity, 17, 63, 65, 69
   and national identity, 123, 130–1
   privileging of, 28, 30, 33, 60, 83
   as proximate sense, 76
   and race, 37, 71, 72–3, 131, 143n39
   and religious expression, 25, 61–3, 64
   and social policy, 65, 67, 68, 69
   and tactility, 111
   and violence, 9
   and women, 32, 66
smellscapes, 60, 69, 73

Smilor, Raymond, 52–3, 136n12
Smith, Jeffrey Chipps, 64
social history, 7, 8, 16, 59, 129, 133n2
Socrates, 42, 60
sound, history of, 42
South Africa, 56
South America, 26, 30, 56
South Carolina, 36, 111
Sterne, Jonathan, 55
Stevens, Scott Manning, 110
street lighting, 25–6, 38
sugar, 79, 83–4, 119, 124
sumptuary law, 16, 77, 83, 105
supermarkets, 126–8
surveillance, 7, 25–6, 34, 67, 95
Sutton, David, 87
Swislocki, Mark S., 88
synesthesia, 9, 30
Synnott, Anthony, 29, 59, 78, 112, 136n10, 141n21
Syria, 60

tasting, 3, 7, 18, 94
   association with women, 32
   and class, 24, 82–3, 89–90, 104, 108, 120–5
   consumption of, 85–7, 90
   and creation of knowledge, 90–1
   eroticism of, 127–8
   and food culture, 79–87, 90
   geography of, 78–9
   history of, 3, 7, 75, 138n30
   marginalization of, 8, 9, 28–9, 41, 76, 77, 81
   and medicine, 141n21
   and modernity, 97
   and national identity, 87–9, 150n31
   privileging of, 10
   as proximate sense, 2, 18
   and race, 37
   religious aspects of, 64, 78, 98–9
   as social force, 7, 76
technology, history of, 7, 133n2, 136n12
Thomas, Keith, 104–5

Thompson, Emily, 54
Thuillier, Guy, 122
tongues, 28, 75, 81, 85, 90–1, 123, 125, 127
Toporkov, Andrei, 38
touching, 1, 8
   and modernity, 95
   and notions of ownership, 96, 114
   public consumption of, 24, 115–16
   as religious expression, 97–9
   taboo of, 108, 112
Tourgee, Albion W., 36
transgression, 25, 27, 32, 59, 111
Tyndale-Biscoe, C. E., 111

United States, 5, 35, 49, 70–1, 74, 84, 102, 116, 126
urban space, 25, 35
urbanization, 1, 25, 26, 52, 66, 82, 90
U.S. Supreme Court, 36

van Ruusbroec, Jan, 98
Vazsonyi, Nicholas, 49
violence, 15, 42, 99, 101–2
vision, *see* seeing
visual distancing, 33
visual space, 11
visual studies, 19, 21
visualism, 10, 11, 13, 23–4, 33

von Goethe, Johann Wolfgang, 100, 129

Wagner, Wilhelm Richard, 49
Walkerton, Ontario, 90–1
Washington, George, 107
whiteness, 5, 35–7, 51, 55–7, 65, 70–3, 85–6, 89, 101, 109, 126
William of Auxerre, 78, 99
Woolf, D.R., 33
women, 27, 127
   and aurality, 45, 51
   as caregivers, 101
   history of, 4, 122
   labor of, 85
   and medicine, 33, 101
   and olfaction, 66
   and seeing, 76
   and sensorial discrimination, 32
   and sight, 76
   and tasting, 88
   and touch, 96–7, 108
   work of, 85, 109
Wu, Yunchu, 88

York Archaeological Trust, 120

Zeigler, Peter, 35, 37
Zimbabwe, 73
Zulus, 56
Zwingli, Huldrych, 64

Printed in Dunstable, United Kingdom